Communicating Wo

M000301964

This volume explores the conditions under which women are empowered, and feel entitled, to make the health decisions that are best for them. At its core, it illuminates how the most basic element of communication, voice, has been summarily suppressed for entire groups of women when it comes to control of their own sexuality, reproductive lives, and health. By giving voice to these women's experiences, the book shines a light on ways to improve health communication for women.

Bringing together personal narratives, key theory and literature, and original qualitative and quantitative studies, the book provides an in-depth comparative picture of how and why women's health varies for distinct groups of women. Organized into four parts—historical influences on patient and provider perceptions, breast cancer the silence and the shame, make it taboo: mothering, reproduction, and motherhood, and sex, sexuality, relational health, and womanhood.

Annette Madlock Gatison, Ph.D., is an Associate Professor at Southern Connecticut State University, USA. Her forthcoming work for 2015 includes *Embracing the Pink Identity: Breast Cancer Culture, Faith Talk and the Myth of the Strong Black Women,* Lexington Books; *The Pink and the Black Experience: Lies that Make Us Suffer in Silence and Cost Us Our Lives,* an article for Women's Studies in Communication; and "Body Politics Strategies for Inclusiveness: A Case Study of the National Breast Cancer Coalition," chapter in *Contexts for the Dark Side of Communication.*

Routledge Research in Health Communication

Communicating Women's Health

Social and Cultural Norms that Influence Health Decisions

Edited by
Annette Madlock Gatison

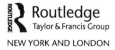

Routledge
Taylor & Francis Group

NEW YORK AND LONDON

First published 2016
by Routledge
711 Third Avenue, New York, NY 10017

and by Routledge
2 Park Square, Milton Park, Abingdon, Oxon OX14 4RN

First issued in paperback 2017

Routledge is an imprint of the Taylor & Francis Group, an informa business

Library of Congress Cataloging-in-Publication Data

Communicating women's health: social and cultural norms that influence health decisions / [edited] by Annette Madlock Gatison.
  p.; cm. — (Routledge research in health communication; 1)
Includes bibliographical references and index.
  I. Madlock Gatison, Annette, editor. II. Series: Routledge research in health communication; 1.
  [DNLM: 1. Women's Health. 2. Cultural Characteristics. 3. Health Communication. 4. Health Status Disparities. 5. Patient Participation. 6. Sexism. WA 309.1]
  RA778
  613'.04244—dc23   2015026738

ISBN 13: 978-0-8153-8649-0 (pbk)
ISBN 13: 978-1-138-84161-1 (hbk)

Typeset in Sabon
by codeMantra

This work is dedicated to women and their families everywhere.

Contents

Introduction

Social, Cultural Norms and Women's Health

Annette Madlock Gatison

In 2002, the Institute of Medicine published *Unequal Treatment: Confronting Racial and Ethnic Disparities in Health Care*, which reported that racial and ethnic minorities experience a lower quality of healthcare than nonminorities, even when they have income and insurance. That report pointed to stereotyping and bias within the healthcare system as the primary culprit and made recommendations about developing culturally competent healthcare as the fundamental way to reduce health disparities. Since then, cultural competency in health communication has become the touchstone for targeted health communication and disease prevention efforts for women and minorities. Unfortunately, this goal will never be achieved unless we hear from the women who continue to fall through the cracks of the still-broken healthcare system. Indeed, in the 21st century, there remain social and cultural norms that manifest themselves via institutional and interpersonal barriers to effective health communication along the lines of race, class, gender, ethnicity, and sexuality that unduly impact women as a group. These social and cultural norms are defined as a pattern of behavior in a particular group, community, or culture, accepted as normal and to which an individual is expected to conform.

Communicating Women's Health is an edited collection that explores how different social locations give rise to beliefs about health, how health concerns are expressed or suppressed, who should be treated and for what, and the conditions under which women are empowered, and feel entitled, to make the health decisions that are best for them. At its core the book illuminates how the most basic element of communication, voice, has been summarily suppressed for entire groups of women when it comes to their mental and physical health, control of their own sexuality and reproductive lives, and their safety. By giving voice to these women's experiences and contextualizing them within multidisciplinary theoretical and contextual frameworks, *Communicating Women's Health* shines a light on ways to improve health communication and elements of the healthcare system itself.

Communicating Women's Health contains original chapters from researchers, advocates, and allies across many disciplines and areas of expertise. Bringing together personal narratives, key theory and literature, and the reporting of original qualitative and quantitative studies, the book provides an in-depth comparative picture of how women's health varies for distinct groups of women, and explains why this variation occurs. Readers discern similarities and differences in women's experiences across a range of health topics, gaining familiarity with the breadth of research techniques used to understand women's health and the contexts that produce patterned, as well as unique, experiences.

The anthology has a thematic organization with Section One, *Historical Influences on Patient and Provider Perceptions*, serving as the introduction and setting the tone for the collection. **Chapter One**, "Voices from the Past: Understanding the Impact of Historical Discrimination on Today's Healthcare System" introduces us to the history of medical discrimination and wrongful treatment that created an environment for institutionalized silencing and self-silencing that influences patient behavior in our current healthcare system.

Chapter Two, "The Culture of Medicine: A Critical Auto-Ethnography of My Encounter with the Healthcare System," speaks to the behavior of healthcare providers related to their training and personal perceptions of "the other," as seen through the eyes of a medical doctor who had become a chronically ill patient. Studies have identified a host of healthcare disparities and demonstrated how people of color tend to be disproportionately affected. Using autoethnography and drawing on Black feminist epistemology, the author identifies and locates the intersecting forms of oppression that continue to marginalize African peoples along race, class, and gender lines within the healthcare system. She describes her experience of lupus, allowing readers to witness her journey from diagnosis to a hospitalization that would change how she practices medicine. The implications of this revealing analysis are that healthcare providers must become fully engaged with how structures of knowledge interact with language, culture, and spirituality as they relate to healing and human development.

Section Two, *Breast Cancer, the Silence and the Shame,* provides an alternative view to the social norms associated with what it means to be a breast cancer survivor and discusses the rhetoric of indoctrination into pink ribbon culture, while silencing those who know that "survivorship" is not a part of their future. **Chapter Three**, "Pink Is for (Survivor) Girls: Late-stage Breast Cancer, Silence, and Pink Ribbon Culture," exposes the dominant "survivor" discourse surrounding breast cancer, which acts as a disciplinary mechanism that encourages conformity to a specific set of practices, while silencing diverse experiences and concealing the social, cultural, and political facets underlying those experiences. Highlighting the importance of addressing the Third Persona (the absent person) constructed through a rhetoric of silence, the missing story in breast cancer culture is the tale told by women diagnosed with late-stage or metastasized breast cancer.

Chapter Four, "Breast Cancer and Shame," addresses the pink ribbon movement and its original desire to remove stigma from breast cancer, while some of its aspects perpetuate shame. This chapter directs attention to the sponsors of women's breast healthcare who show support for this movement and are therefore implicated in the movement's shaming. The author outlines potential effects of pink ribbon artifacts on the patient's conceptions of self. By problematizing the pink ribbon's presence in one location of women's breast healthcare, a patient waiting area connected to a mammography imaging room, the author extends current critiques of the pink ribbon movement and calls for those engaged in women's breast healthcare to consider the implications of their support of the pink ribbon.

The next four chapters make up the third section, *Make It Taboo: Motherhood, Mothering, and Reproduction,* and are indicative of sociocultural norms surrounding womanhood, mothering, and reproduction from varied and distinct cultural perspectives. **Chapter Five,** "Giving Voice to Women's Childbirth Preferences," discusses current medical and cultural practices in the United States that limit women's choices in labor and delivery. It addresses the current birthing options available and promoted by obstetricians and hospitals (i.e., Cesarean surgery), pharmaceuticals administered during labor and delivery, and hospital policies stipulating compulsory treatment, such as medication for pain management and continuous electronic fetal monitoring, that tend to tip the scale toward a medical model and away from natural childbirth, despite women's preferences.

Chapter Six, "Hush, Little Baby, Don't Say a Word: Nursing Narratives through New Media," is coauthored by a mother and daughter, and reveals the fragmented transgenerational connections among women as they surface in online discussions of breastfeeding taboos. This analysis foregrounds the limitations and possibilities of new media in the documentation and exchange of breastfeeding experiences and, in doing so, proposes innovative methods for studying taboos related to women's health issues.

Chapter Seven, "What Do Prenatal and Postnatal Women Discuss with Their Healthcare Providers?" provides an analysis of the Los Angeles Mommy and Baby (LAMB) 2007 survey, which examines the similarities and differences in doctor–patient communications for Chinese and Caucasian women during their prepregnancy, prenatal, and postnatal physician visits. The authors argue that because the medical system is oriented toward a Caucasian "majority" population, it may not fully address a minority population's health needs that are rooted in their particular cultural values.

Chapter Eight, "Japanese Women's Suicide and Depression under the Panopticon," discusses the patriarchal family system in Japanese culture, called *ie*, which forces women to neglect themselves and their own families in favor of the families of their husband. The image of the ideal *ie* woman contributes to conditions that favor suicide among Japanese women. Japanese historical stories and modern media both present suicide as a courageous act signifying the ultimate self-sacrifice. Rather than seeking outside help, women who experience depression (*utsu*) as a result of patriarchal family relations tend to adhere to this cultural myth. In this chapter, the author shares the stories of two women, both victims of *utsu*, who committed suicide after years of trying to be the ideal *ie* wife/mother in a strict family environment.

The final section, *Sexuality, Relational Health, and Womanhood,* opens with **Chapter Nine**, "Sexual and Relational Health Messages for Women Who Have Sex with Women (WSW)." This discussion of the relatively low risk and low rates of sexually transmitted infections resulting from female-to-female sexual contact contributes to the general misperception that women who have sex with women (WSW) do not need safe sex education. However, these women are still at risk for bacterial, viral, and protozoal infections that have long-term health consequences, such as human papillomavirus (HPV), which can be transmitted through female-to-female sexual contact. In addition, many women who have sex with women also have a history, or current practice, of having sex with men, thereby increasing their risk of contracting or transmitting a sexually transmitted infection. This chapter contextualizes data from an online survey and a content analysis of sexuality texts targeted at WSW to highlight the cultural, political, and relational factors that influence sex communication for this group.

Chapter Ten, "Does This Mean I'm Dirty: The Complexities of Choice in Women's Conversations about HPV Vaccinations." This study explores the collective narratives of 17 women to reveal the mediated strategies that pressure women into particular health options. It explores the complex, sometimes contradictory, concerns of women regarding HPV vaccination and the factors that influence their decisions to have the vaccination. Stories of "testing negative for HPV" illuminate how women contribute to larger understandings of public health and, therefore, influence the ethical deliberation and societal choices considered among health leaders.

Chapter Eleven, "American Menstruation Rhetoric as Sanitized Discourse: Iterating Stigma Through Print Advertisements." According to the author's analysis, stigmatized communication and discourses of repression surrounding menstruation have become accepted ideology in American consumer culture. The author uses Foucault's theory of the repressive hypothesis as a lens to analyze advertisements in women's magazines that help to shape public discourse about menstruation by using body shame and taboo to sell feminine hygiene products.

Closing with **Chapter Twelve**, "Voicing Women's Abortion Stories within Larger Cultural Narratives," the author shares interviews with 14 women of varying backgrounds to reveal how facets of identity (race, class, age) impact both the experience of abortion and women's broader reproductive health experiences. These facets are tied together within the broader cultural narratives about agency and self-empowerment, self-expression, power and privilege, social support, and cautionary tales about careless women.

There are many personal, cultural, and political complexities involved in communicating about women's health that create silence. Some of those complexities are shared here in hopes that the attention to this detail can begin to create an atmosphere of sound—the sound of women comfortably talking about their mental and physical healthcare needs and receiving the message that it is safe for them to do so.

Section I

Historical Influences on Patient and Provider Perceptions

1   Voices from the Past

Understanding the Impact of Historical Discrimination on Today's Healthcare System

Katie Love

Echoes from the Past

Healthcare has a painful history of discrimination and wrongful treatment, leading to changes in patients' behaviors when interacting with the healthcare system of today. These behaviors include self-silencing through passing behaviors (talking and acting like a member of a majority group, such as a lesbian passing as a heterosexual person) and not following doctor/provider advice, or a silencing by the healthcare system through the prevention of diversity among providers, covert discrimination, and manifesting as health disparities. Unfortunately, this silencing process creates major barriers to holistic patient care because a complete understanding is concealed by the patient or is presumed by providers. There is an institutionalized silencing and self-silencing of women of color, lesbians, and women with mental health problems.

Goffman (1963) described the phenomenon of passing as the adoption of behaviors, appearance, and attitudes of the dominant culture, but he originally proposed the term as subconscious and unintentionally conforming to social desirability. For many groups, passing behaviors are developed consciously to also avoid harm, discrimination, and being denied access, as well as gaining the power and privilege bestowed on the dominant cultures (Ginsberg, 1996; Hostert, 2007). In order to navigate the healthcare system, people who have been historically mistreated may perceive the need to develop passing skills in order to get care. In healthcare, these passing behaviors can include adopting the language, communication style, and appearance that will make the person seem to be a member of the dominant group. This charade also includes choosing not to disclose one's identity at all if it is possible to hide (such as sexual orientation, mental illness, or religion). Some may also develop perfectionist behaviors to prove equality. For example, a woman may need to perform much better at her job then her male counterpart to break through the proverbial glass ceiling.

Not all women from within a group can pass in the same ways. Lighter-skinned women or people with European physical characteristics can pass as White in appearance as well as behaviors, but darker-skinned women can only adopt behaviors. A woman with a physical disability may also not be able to pass as able-bodied, whereas other people with physical restrictions such as blindness may be able to pass as sighted persons. Other groups are not visibly in a disenfranchised group unless they choose to disclose it, such as sexual orientation, religion, or mental illness. This group is especially important because nondisclosure could result in inappropriate care, but because such differences are nonvisible, the provider cannot rely on an external cue. Therefore, the individual can successfully self-silence if the provider does not supply a space or sense of safety for this person to disclose.

Discrimination and mistreatment is not just a part of healthcare's history but continues today in new forms. Systemic discrimination exists in modern healthcare because of a complex collision of reasons, including lack of diversity among providers, professional socialization to the majority culture, and the stereotyping of certain diseases to particular groups of people. Because of this history and because of modern risks, women often choose to not disclose their background. This is especially true of women who can pass as belonging to other groups, such as a Wiccan/Pagan woman being able to pass as Christian. In this situation, passing prevents immediate harm, but if the provider is unaware of the person's religion, health teaching may be inappropriate, practices not integrated, and resources not discussed—and ultimately poor care is provided. Therefore it is the responsibility of care providers to learn about people, our shared history, and to create safe and open spaces for all voices to speak.

Understanding Healthcare's History

Events, both major publicized events and innumerable anecdotal events, have negatively shaped the cultural consciousness of disenfranchised people surrounding healthcare and its providers. America's history of disenfranchised peoples coming into contact with healthcare has included substandard treatment, no treatment, or unethical treatment, and this continues today through the epidemic of health disparities. Therefore, it is important to understand the impact of healthcare's history with the Tuskegee experiments, forced sterilization, and abuses of gay and lesbians, people, as well as with disabilities and mental health issues in institutional settings: this history has undeniably created mistrust, fear, and anger among many groups in the United States. People understand this as a part of their group's history, as their present, and as something to guard against in the future through self-silencing.

The Tuskegee syphilis experiment is likely the most well-known abuse of research subjects and specifically of African Americans. The experiment lasted from 1932 to 1972, and involved a group of 399 poor African American men with syphilis who were untreated in order for researchers to study the natural progression of the disease. Twenty-eight of the original 399 men had died of syphilis, 100 died of related complications, 40 of their wives were infected, and 19 of their children were born with congenital syphilis. The Tuskegee experiment left a "legacy of mistrust" for African Americans, mistrust of both research and of the healthcare community (Bhopal, 1998; Birn & Molina, 2005). Tuskegee has come to represent racism in medicine, physician arrogance, misconduct in research, and government abuse of people of color (Gamble, 1997).

Although the Tuskegee syphilis experiment is the most widely cited example of mistreatment in healthcare, the mistreatment and subsequent distrust started long before. Slavery prevented people from receiving any healthcare, so people relied on folk medicine, a trend that continues among many disenfranchised groups today (Kennedy, Mathis, & Woods, 2007). During Reconstruction, White medical schools used people of color and the poor to practice assessment and procedures, and to perform autopsies. This medical attention was promoted as free health care, but as people shared stories of mistreatment, the mistrust grew. Additionally, the stories of "night doctors" or "Klu Klux Doctors," people who robbed graves for cadavers and kidnapped living people of color and the poor for medical schools, reinforced fears of hospitals and healthcare (Clark, 2009). Through segregation, African American people were turned away at White-only hospitals to die on the hospital's doorstep or on the way to a hospital or doctor that would treat them. For women of color, this history is critical to an understanding of why many Black women do not seek healthcare, are resistant to starting drug regimens, to following medical advice, and to bringing in their children for medical care as well (Hine, 1989; Kennedy, Mathis, & Woods, 2007; Patterson, 2009).

Eugenics is another important area of discrimination in the history of healthcare. Eugenics is the selective breeding of people for the best genetic outcome of humanity and was wildly popular in the late 19th and early 20th centuries. Researchers at the time believed that mental illness, poverty, low intelligence (feeblemindedness), physical disability, and crime could all be eradicated through the sterilization of people within these groups. Many women were asked about sterilization right after C-sections; some women were unaware of their options and were coerced by physicians and the government who informed them that it was best for them and that sterilization had health benefits (Mass, 1977). Legally, distinctions were also made between the forced sterilization of women in mental institutions and the coercive sterilization of poor and immigrant communities (Birn & Molina, 2005). The criteria for forced sterilization included institutionalized women, but women who had children out of wedlock, were lesbians, or masturbated were sometimes classified as nymphomaniacs and thus were deemed mentally ill as well (Stern, 2005).

Forced or coerced sterilization of institutionalized women, the poor, women of color, and women with limited English proficiency was supported by major societal influencers such as businesspeople, the medical community, research funding, government agencies, and laws. Sterilization was compulsory by law in 30 states and in Puerto Rico until as late as the 1970s when a federal law prohibiting it was established (Birn & Molina, 2005; Mass, 1977). This delay in action has been perceived as evidence of overwhelming support of sterilization, and it has prolonged distrust of the medical system, ultimately resulting in passing behaviors as a form of self-protection to ensure the best care possible. The removal of all reproductive rights among poor women of color is a part of healthcare's history and greatly impacts this group's fear and distrust of the healthcare system (Stern, 2005).

The importance of these events is reflected in the overwhelming distrust of the medical communities, and these events still have relevance to healthcare today. These stories are saddening and often disturbing to healthcare providers who are not aware of this history, and yet although the overt behaviors of the past no longer exist, they have been replaced by more covert forms of bias such as labeling people as noncompliant, uncooperative, or drug-seeking. Health disparities are another way that bias is found, whether it is conscious or subconscious.

Health Disparities

The tensions between stereotypes held by the healthcare providers, society at large, and the historical memory of many disenfranchised groups of women have sustained the health disparity gap and the perceived need for passing behaviors and self-silencing. Today's health disparities show that not all people are treated the same and have the same outcomes despite diagnostic similarities (CDC, 2001; Hebert, Sisk, & Howell, 2008; Smedley, Stith, & Nelson, 2002). Health disparities are differences in the incidence, prevalence, mortality, and burden of diseases and other adverse health conditions that exist among specific population groups in the United States (CDC, 2001). A true health disparity must also control for other issues such as economics (Hebert, Sisk, & Howell, 2008; Betancourt & King, 2003).

For women who need to disclose their identity, these disparities can be particularly difficult to isolate. If one chooses to pass as a heterosexual, and the healthcare provider presumes heterosexuality, then patients can be misdiagnosed or underdiagnosed (Simkin, 1998). Lesbian women who choose to disclose their sexual identity in the course of their obstetric/midwifery care have met with overfocusing on their sexuality, assumptions, stereotypes, homophobic prejudice, and discrimination (Wilton, 1999; Spidberg, 2007). According to Anderson and Holliday (2004), 85% of gays and lesbians at some time pass as straight. Despite this high number, there is growing mental health research that now marginalizes LGBTs who are not "out." In this same study, closeted people were often labeled as having low self-esteem, poor self-image, latent homophobia, poor interpersonal relationships, the inability to give/receive love, depression, and self-hatred (Anderson & Holliday, 2004). This forms a kind of problem for an LGBT patient who they may be stigmatized for disclosure, but also pathologized for nondisclosure (Anderson & Holliday, 2004; Kanuha, 1997; Cain, 1991). Both of these scenarios place the burden on the patient, and place them in a self-defending position regardless of the approach chosen.

The Culture of Healthcare

The expected norms of healthcare reflect the ideas of the dominant group, which are accepted by patients, staff, and provider educational programs. Therefore, in order for people to successfully navigate the healthcare system, they must know what they are expected to do, how to do it, and to be aware that they will be evaluated by these behaviors. Although disenfranchised groups recognize that the dominant norms are different from the norms of their group identity, giving voice to the problem is also speaking against the dominant group. In healthcare this is seen every day when patients nod in understanding to concepts they do not understand, when they agree with a treatment plan that is inappropriate to their own culture, or when they simply choose to remain silent and pass as being from a different group than their own.

In addition to the behaviors of patients interacting with the healthcare system, there is a professional socialization to the norms of the dominant culture. The normed dominant culture within the healthcare system is so entrenched that it is viewed as 'professional' behavior rather than cultural behavior. Healthcare students with identities different from those of the dominant culture (White, male, middle class, able-bodied, heterosexual) often struggle in their education due to the professional socialization process (Love, 2008).

After the 2002 Institute of Medicine report, the United States government and the Office of Minority Health developed standards for Culturally and Linguistically Appropriate Services (CLAS) (Smedley, Stith, & Nelson, 2002). The American Nurses Association, the American Academy of Nurses, and the Transcultural Nursing Society all have culturally competent care as a goal and a priority. In addition to the large body of evidence-based practice suggesting ways of improving cultural competence, healthcare centers across the United States have changed mission statements, bylaws, and organizational standards to support culturally competent care.

Despite this documented focus, the actualization of cultural practice and cultural education presents several problems (Sullivan, 2004). Culture is taught as other, meaning that American White and dominant culture is not taught but is assumed as the location of the students, and so "culture" then becomes that which is different from oneself (Allen, 2006; Carberry, 1998; Markey & Tilki, 2007). Students learn generalizations of cultural groups to be used as a blueprint for making nursing care decisions (Allen, 2006; Dreher & MacNaughton, 2002). This is problematic in creating stereotypes and assumes that all people from a particular culture subscribe to all its practices and traditions as well.

Culture is often taught in a way that portrays it as static and ahistorical (Hassouneh, 2006; Love, 2008; Markey & Tilki, 2007). The lack of anti-discrimination education in healthcare ignores the social structures caused by inequity and oppression that maintain the health disparities seen today (Hassouneh, 2006; Markey & Tilki, 2007; Pollock Kossman, 2003; Zinn, 2003). In addition to gender identity, people of color, people who speak English as a second language, are homosexual, transgendered, or have mental or physical disabilities must be aware of the expected professional behaviors and are socialized to expect the same of their patients and of their peers within the healthcare community.

When schools are organized in an ethnocentric manner, students from the dominant groups stand to benefit the most (Hassouneh-Phillips & Beckett, 2003; McQueen & Zimmerman, 2004). In order for professional passing to take place, the dominant culture must be chosen as a professional identity. This is true across the healthcare system. The medical model has long been associated with masculine characteristics, being viewed as rationality over intuition, diagnosis over holism, and professional distance over emotional and spiritual interconnectedness. In medicine, many speculated that medical practice would change as women entered the profession. In the modern United States, there are equal numbers of men and women graduating from medical schools, some graduating more women, yet the status quo of the medical model in practice has been maintained. Although it is unclear if women have exhibited passing behaviors to meet the expectations of the medical profession, it is undeniable that the masculine (not necessarily male) characteristics and perspectives are a medical cultural norm. These characteristics are expected not only from the rest of the healthcare community, but also from society at large.

Detriments of Self-Silencing

One of the problems with passing behaviors is that the woman who is trying to pass is often doing so unsuccessfully. There is often language that is not understood, cues that are missed, and people putting themselves at risk when they try to "guess" at the expected actions/behaviors. Although it is common for any layperson interacting with healthcare to resist asking questions or asking for clarification of providers, the problems are magnified for people outside of the dominant cultural group because they may not have a context for understanding what was discussed, not have the English language proficiency to know how to seek answers at a later time, or miss opportunities to receive culturally relevant health teaching.

Currently, it is the patient's responsibility to admit that he or she does not know what something is or to provide information about his or her culture to get clearer information. This requires such patients to admit that they do not understand something, to confront a person of perceived power (which may be culturally inappropriate), or to be aware that the information they are being given may have a cultural impact at all. This issue is especially important for people who do not visibly belong to a discriminated-against group such as LGBT, who do not have mental illnesses or disabilities, and who have some religious identity. Choosing to disclose this information may result in being treated differently, if not being subjected to outright discrimination.

Among people from the LGBT community, passing behaviors often include pretending to have heterosexual relationships and going along with assumptions such as the gender of a partner, reporting engaging in the sexual behaviors anticipated by the provider, or being unable to have same-sex partners present during treatment. When considering that the healthcare provider is not aware of the health needs of their patients without this information, there are potentially long-term risks associated with these passing behaviors.

Another example involves people with disabilities in the healthcare setting, who often attempt to pass as able-bodied people. They guess at the meaning of words, and they overstate their ability to perform a task (such as self administering insulin or changing a dressing). Grue and Laerum (2002; Cain, 1991) explored the passing behaviors of mothers with disabilities and found that since the stereotypes were that people with disabilities are care receivers and not caregivers and that children may be removed if these mothers are not seen to be "normal mothers," the desire to pass as mothering normally was great. These mothers felt tremendous pressure to present a perfect performance of motherhood, to not have their children seen as being their helpers, and even to prove their gender and motherhood. These are all experiences and behaviors that able-bodied mothers never need to think about in their daily lives.

What's Next?

The reasons that people may enact passing behaviors, either consciously or unconsciously, are most often rooted in fear. Understanding the historical context is critical to understanding why a group of people may act with distrust when encountering a healthcare provider. Even for people who choose to pass in opposition to stereotypes, the resistance is based on the historical oppression faced by this group. It can be empowering to pass, as it shifts the power differential toward the individual choosing the identity they will be judged by (Cain, 1991; Hostert, 2007, White, 2006). Healthcare providers can learn more about the history of oppressed groups, giving them better perspective about the attitudes and behaviors of a group and helping them learn how to provide more supportive and validating interactions.

Bias in the United States has changed from overt to covert, which pushes issues from social structure to an individual issue. Colorblind practice erases color (and the other identities), and therefore nondominant identities seem to disappear. This obscures and undermines women's experiences of racism, sexism, classism, homophobia, and discrimination, and allows a labeling of women from nondominant groups who speak out as angry, problematic, violent, and lazy (Collins, 1990, 2004). "Colorblindness" is therefore offensive because the message is that identity does not matter, but "colorblindness" is actualized as treating everyone as being from the dominant culture of White, middle-class, Christian, able-bodied, and heterosexual.

Healthcare providers learn passing culture in school and may adopt these dominant behaviors and beliefs as normal, not just for themselves but also for their patients. The call for more diversity among healthcare providers cannot simply be done without support of the cultural behaviors, communication styles, and lifestyles of people from all backgrounds. Allen (2006) describes the ideology guiding many schools in diversity education as "add color and stir" (p. 67). Schools accomplish this by believing cultural competence improves simply by increasing clinical experiences with people of color, adding people of color to faculty and student bodies, and courses to the curriculum. This analogy can easily be extended to all groups of people different from oneself, as 'add diversity and stir,' and does not allow for critical analysis of social structures that create problems. Nor does it allow for reflection of oppression experiences by patients or students from nondominant groups. It also assumes that diversity can be achieved simply by having a person who belongs to a particular group, but does not acknowledge that the individual may not identify with this group (Allen, 2006; Dreher & MacNaughton, 2002). Therefore, more needs to be done to support difference, identity, and culture in schools for healthcare providers and to include experiences and discussions where such differences can be accessed and supported by even a student body that is homogeneous of dominant groups.

Conclusion

Healthcare is taken for granted by many privileged people whose identities make it an expectation to access healthcare when it is needed; for these people, care will not involve questioning of one's lifestyle, and testing, diagnosis, and treatment will all have the patient's individual needs altruistically in mind. For many Americans, this is simply not the case.

People may adopt passing behaviors subconsciously, as Goffman suggested, as the influence of social desirability and cultural norming invades the psyche. For some it is a matter of self-protection, of protecting their families and children, and of fears of discrimination and mistreatment. In the best cases, choosing to pass as a person from the dominant groups can be an empowering experience rooted in the intent to express oneself as one chooses rather than as others may project on to them, to bring public awareness to the presence of a group of people, and to take control of situations that may result in discrimination to prevent such outcomes (White, 2006).

Silencing in healthcare, regardless of the intentions behind it can have very negative consequences that may result in missed opportunities, in mis-diagnosis, and in maintaining the status quo of a dominant healthcare culture. Currently, the responsibility to address these issues is on the patients and the disenfranchised women, but that needs to change. More support for cultural and subcultural expression needs to be given in the academic preparation of healthcare providers. Providers need to understand and learn about the cultural context and history of healthcare from the perspective of disenfranchised women. The discrimination experiences of different groups of people today also need to be understood to alter the approach and perspectives of the healthcare providers when working with people from non-dominant groups. Finally, the medical model and the Western belief that color-blindness and neutrality are healthy, preferred, or even possible need to be removed from the educational system of healthcare providers and from the models that guide learning and knowledge construction. When this occurs, people may be more likely to create the social changes necessary to alter policies, improve access, address health disparities by focusing on the social structures, and of creating safe spaces for the voices of women from all backgrounds.

References

Allen, D. (2006). Whiteness and difference in nursing. *Nursing Philosophy, 7*, 65–78.

ANA. (2006) *Nurses renew push for passage of nursing shortage legislation 2001.* Retrieved from http://www.nursingworld.org/pressrel/2001/pr1204.htm.

Anderson, S., & M. Holliday. (2004). Normative passing in the lesbian community: An exploratory study. *Journal of Gay and Lesbian Social Services, 17*(3), 25–38.

Ashton, P. (1996). The concept of activity. In *Vygotsky in the classroom. Mediated literacy instruction and assessment.* New York: Longman Publishers.

Betancourt, J., & K. King. (2003). Unequal treatment: The Institute of Medicine report and its public health implications. *Public Health Reports, 118*, 287–292.

Bhopal, R. (1998) Spectre of Racism in Health and Health Care: Lessons from History and the United States. *British Medical Journal, 316*(7149), 1970–1973.

Birn, A., & N. Molina. (2005). In the name of public health. *American Journal of Public Health, 95*(7), 1095–1098.

Cain, R. (1991). Stigma management and gay identity development. *Social Work, 36*(1), 67–73.

Campinha-Bacote, Josephina. (2007). Becoming culturally competent in ethnic psychopharmacology. *Journal of Psychosocial Nursing, 45*(9), 27–36.

Carberry, C. (1998). Contesting competency: Cultural safety in advanced practice. *Collegian, 5*(4), 9–13.

CDC. (2007). *Health disparities affecting minorities: African Americans 2001.* Retrieved from http://www.cdc.gov.cancer/healthdisparities/statistics/ethnic.htm.

Census, U.S. Bureau of. (2006). *School enrollment population survey 2000.* Retrieved from http://www.askcensus.gov.

Clark, P. (2009). Prejudice and the medical profession: A five-year update. *Journal of Law, Medicine, and Ethics, 37*(1), 118–133.

Coates, R. (2004). If a tree falls in the wilderness: Reparations, academic silences, and social justice. *Social Forces, 83*(2), 841–864.

Collins, P. H. (1990). *Black feminist thought: Knowledge, consciousness, and the politics of empowerment.* New York: Routledge.

Collins, P. H. (2004). *Black sexual politics.* New York: Routledge.

Dreher, M., & N. MacNaughton. (2002). Cultural competence in nursing: Foundation or fallacy? *Nursing Outlook, 50*, 181–186.

Freire, P. (1973). *Education for critical consciousness.* New York: Seabury.

Gamble, V. N. (1997). Under the shadow of Tuskegee: African Americans and health care. *American Journal of Public Health, 87*(11), 1773–1779.

Ginsberg, E. (1996). *Passing and the fictions of identity.* Durham, NC: Duke University Press.

Giroux, H. (2003). Critical theory and educational practice. In *The critical pedagogy reader*, edited by A. Darder, M. Baltodano, and R. Torres. New York: Routledge Falmer.

Giroux, H. (1988). *Teachers as intellectuals: Toward a critical pedagogy of learning.* Westport, CT: Bergin & Garvey.

Goffman, E. (1963). *Stigma: Notes on the management of spoiled identity.* Englewood Cliffs, NJ: Prentice Hall.

Gramsci, A. (1971). *Selections from the prison notebooks.* New York: International Publishers.

Grue, L., & K. Laerum. (2002). "Doing motherhood": Some experiences of mothers with physical disabilities. *Disability and Society, 17*(6), 671–683.

Haigh, C., & M. Johnson. (2007). Attitudes and values of nurse educators: An international survey. *Berkley Electronic Press, 4*(1), 1–11.

Hassouneh, D. (2006). Anti-racist pedagogy: Challenges faced by faculty of color in predominantly White schools of nursing. *Journal of Nursing Education, 45*(7), 255–263.

Hassouneh-Phillips, D., & A. Beckett. (2003). An education in racism. *Journal of Nursing Education, 42*(6), 258–265.

Hebert, P., Sisk, J. & Howell, E. (2008). When does a difference become a disparity? *Conceptualizing racial and ethnic disparities in health. 27*(2):374–82. doi: 10.1377/hlthaff.27.2.374.

Hine, D. C. (1989). *Black women in white: Racial conflict and cooperation in the nursing profession 1890–1950.* Indianapolis: Indiana University Press.

Hostert, A. (2007). *Passing: A strategy to dissolve identities and remap difference.* Translated by C. Marciasini. Cranbury, NJ: Rosemont Publishing.

Jordan, J. (1996). Rethinking race/attraction in nursing programs: A hermeneutic inquiry. *Journal of Professional Nursing, 12*(6), 382–390.

Kanuha, V. (1997). Stigma, identity, and passing: How lesbians and gay men of color construct and manage stigmatized identity in social interaction. Unpublished doctoral dissertation, University of Washington, Seattle.

Katz, A. (2009). Gay and lesbian patients with cancer. *Oncology Nursing Forum, 36*(2), 203–207.

Kennedy, B., Mathis, C., & A. Woods. (2007). African Americans and their mistrust of the health care system: Healthcare for diverse populations. *Journal of Cultural Diversity, 14*(2), 56–62.

Ladson-Billings, G. (1995). Toward a theory of culturally relevant pedagogy. *American Educational Research Journal, 32*(3), 465–491.

Lea, A. (1994). Nursing in today's multicultural society: A transcultural perspective. *Journal of Advanced Nursing, 20*(2), 307–313.

Lipscomb, L. (1975). *Socialization factors in the development of Black children's racial self-esteem.* Paper presented at the Annual Meeting of the American Sociological Association, San Francisco, CA.

Love, K. A. (2008). Case studies of critical first-year science teachers. Doctoral Dissertation. Paper AAI3323502, Education, University of Connecticut, Storrs, CT.

Lynn, M. (2006). Race, culture, and the education of African-Americans. *Educational Theory, 56*(1), 107–119.

Markey, K., & M. Tilki. (2007). Racism in nursing education: A reflective journey. *British Journal of Nursing, 16*(7), 390–395.

Mass, B. (1977). Puerto Rico: A case study of population control. *Latina American Perspectives, 4*(66), 66–81.

Mathews, M. (1996). Vygotsky in writing: Children using language to learn and learning from children's language what to teach. In *Vygotsky in the classroom. Mediated literacy instruction and assessment.* New York: Longman.

McQueen, L., & L. Zimmerman. (2004). The role of historically Black colleges and universities in the inclusion and education of Hispanic nursing students. *American Black Nurses Foundation Journal, 15*(3), 51–54.

O'Hanlan, K., Dibble, S., Hagan, J., & R. Davis. (2004). Advocacy for women's health should include lesbian health. *Journal of Women's Health, 13*(2), 227–239.

Patterson, A. (2009). Germs and Jim Crow: The impact of microbiolodgy on public health policies in progressive era American south. *Journal of History and Biology, 45*, 529–559.

Pollock Kossman, S. (2003). Student and faculty perceptions of nursing education culture and its impact on minority students. Doctor of Philosophy, Department of Educational Administration and Foundations, Illinois State University.

Rather, M. (1994). Schooling for oppression: A critical hermeneutical analysis of the lived experience of the returning RN student. *Journal of Nursing Education, 33*(6), 263–271.

Rogge, M., & M. Greenwald. (2004). Obesity, stigma, and civilized oppression. *Advances in Nursing Science, 27*(4), 301–315.

Schulman, K., Berlin, J., Harless, W., Kerner, J., Sistrunk, S., & B. Gersh. (1999). The effect of race and sex on physicians' recommendations for cardiac catherization. *New England Journal of Medicine, 340*, 618–626.

Simkin, R. (1998). Not all of your patients are straight. *Canadian Medical Association Journal, 1*(59), 370–375.

Spidberg, B. (2007). Vulnerable and strong: Lesbian women encountering maternity care. *Journal of Advanced Nursing, 60*(5), 478–486.

Stern, A. (2005). Sterilized in the name of public health: Race, immigration, and reproduction control in modern California. *American Journal of Public Health, 95*(7), 1128–1138.

Sullivan, L. (2004). *Missing persons: Minorities in health professions. A report of the Sullivan Commission on diversity in the healthcare workforce.* Retrieved from http://www.picosearch.com/cgi-bmts.pl.

Tarca, K. (2005). Colorblind in control: The risks of resisting difference amid demographic change. *Educational Studies, 38*(2), 99–120.

Tashiro, C. (2005a). The meaning of race in health care and research—Part 1: The impact of history. *Pediatric Nursing, 31*(3), 208–210.

Tashiro, C. (2005b). The meaning of race in healthcare research—part 2: Emerging research. *Pediatric Nursing, 31*(4), 305–308.

Tong, R. (1989). *Feminist thought: A comprehensive introduction.* Boulder, CO: Westview Press.

Waltz, M. (2005). Reading case studies of people with autistic spectrum disorders: A cultural studies approach to issues of disability representation. *Disability and Society, 20*(4), 421–435.

White, A. (2006). Racial and gender attitudes as predictors of feminist activism among self-identified African-American feminists. *Journal of Black Psychology, 32*(4), 455–478.

Wilton, T. (1999). Towards an understanding of the cultural roots of homophobia in order to provide a better midwifery service for lesbian clients. *Midwifery, 15*, 154–164.

World Health Organization. (1973). *Technical Report Series. No. 512.* Washington, DC: Author.

Yoder, M. (1996). Instructional responses to ethnically divers nursing students. *Journal of Nursing Education, 35*(7), 310–315.

Zinn, H. (2003). *A people's history of the United States* New York: HarperCollins.

2 The Culture of Medicine

A Critical Autoethnography of My Encounter with the Healthcare System

Denise Hooks-Anderson and
Reynaldo Anderson

Introduction

The psychological and physical state of individuals suffering from chronic illness is closely linked to their self-identity and dynamically interacts with the social boundaries of the broader society (Clarke & James, 2003). Moreover, an individual's self-identity may go through changes as it reflexively interprets and reinterprets the identification with which others including the 'self' may frame him or her (Clarke & James, 2003). Correspondingly, the training that medical providers receive in regard to power relations in patients' experiences of suffering during treatment is an underappreciated phenomenon. Therefore, to improve patient outcomes and reduce suffering, it is crucial to examine how 'power relations' influence patient experiences of suffering during a treatment for chronic illness. According to De Los Reyes and Mulinari, the elements of race/ethnicity, gender, and class do not operate in isolation, and these constructs inform each other mutually and cooperatively (2005). Furthermore, in relation to 'power relations,' studies have shown in recent years that inequality in healthcare can be associated with stereotypes connected to ethnicity, gender, and lack of resources (Carlsen & Kaarboe, 2010; Malterud, 2010). Also, due to the fact that in relation to suffering there is a correlation between 'power relations' and patient dependency, and how this is related to delivery of care, illness, and quality of life, there is a need to investigate this phenomenon (Eriksson, 2006). For example, according to Morse (2001), there are three stages of suffering: *enduring, emotional suffering*, and *reconciliation*. During the *enduring* stage, patients shut down their emotional reactions and suppress their feelings until a safe environment encourages more insight. The *emotional suffering* stage patients may understand their predicament but are unable to recognize a way out. Finally, when patients reach the point where they can envision a new beginning, they have entered the stage of *reconciliation*. Therefore, it is incumbent to research 'power relations' and inequality in healthcare from an intersectional perspective that creates awareness of different positions of privilege and that examine the historical constructions of power and how these constructs limit the quality of healthcare.

Background

For doctors, it all starts with the first day of the third year of medical school. Medical students at this time are introduced to the inpatient hospital experience. Most students are idealistic, full of vigor and excitement, and are prepared to become a medical apprentice for the next two years. Their future practice of medicine may be determined by those positive or negative experiences that are forthcoming. To understand their experience, one must understand how training hospitals operate. The intern is the physician who does most of the work. He or she is the person who gets the majority of the calls from the nursing staff in regards to the patients. If a medication is needed, the nurse contacts the intern first. This allows the intern to gain experience in making decisions. A more senior resident or attending is also available if questions arise.

The process starts from the initial admitting orders given on behalf of the patient. After the patient is admitted, the senior resident and attending then set the schedule for how the upcoming days will proceed. A time is set when the team will round the next day. For example, if the time is set for 8 am, then this means the intern will need to be ready at least an hour to two hours in advance. The intern is expected to have done all of the prework for the senior resident and attending. Therefore, for the patient this often means that he or she is being awakened at 5:30 or 6:00 am. The intern then meets the other members of the team, discusses his or her findings, develops a plan of care, and then returns to the patient's room with the entire team, possibly six or seven people.

I had been involved in the aforementioned scenario on multiple occasions as a student and resident. Because of that, I am sure my actions were somewhat robotic. And for most of those occasions, I thought the procedure was going well and I was providing outstanding care. However, later, after my own hospitalization, I was thoroughly embarrassed and disgusted with the healthcare system. I was able to pinpoint multiple instances where the healthcare/hospital system had failed.

In 2001, I began having some peculiar symptoms that were not really specific for any particular disorder. I first noticed that I was having night sweats. I did not think much of it. I was also extremely tired, but I was a wife, young mother, and physician. I had multiple reasons to be experiencing fatigue. At my gynecology visit, the doctor insisted on doing a needle aspiration. She believed the lump she found was a cyst. After no aspirate was obtained, she then referred me to a surgeon. The surgeon recommended a biopsy. During the surgery he sent a small sample to the pathologist for a preliminary reading. In the recovery room following the surgery, the surgeon revealed to my husband and me that the sample appeared to be cancer, but more tests would have to be done to be certain. At this point, all I could do was cry. I had only been married four years, had a one-year-old daughter, and had just started my career. My entire life flashed before my eyes. A tiny sample of tissue had potentially altered the course of my existence.

Therefore, 2001 began my entrance into the healthcare system as a chronic disease sufferer with frequent doctor visits, multiple co-pays, expensive medications, and several unanswered questions. I was now experiencing what my patients had been trying to explain to me. I could now relate to the long wait times, prior authorizations for medications, and rude office. I was fortunate to have what was considered "good" health insurance. "Good" health insurance meant that I did not have huge deductibles and it paid for most things. The problem came when I tried to get disability insurance. Disability insurance covers you if for some reason you are unable to work for an extended amount of time. This insurance, short term or long term, will pay you a portion of your salary. Short term would start payment after about 6 weeks of medical leave, and long term would begin at about 3–6 months depending upon the plan.

I quickly found out about preexisting health conditions. Basically, insurance carriers want you to be a no-risk client. If you had any health condition prior to starting their policy, they could potentially deny you coverage or make your rates astronomically higher, as in my case. The insurer could also grant you coverage but exclude your specific disease. This was all prior to the Affordable Care Act. As a resident in training, the business manager of the program advised all of us residents to get disability insurance while we were young and healthy. Very few of us followed the advice. We were barely surviving on our miniscule salaries for basic needs such as housing, transportation, and food. As I started to navigate the healthcare system, I had a unique opportunity to see the system with a different perspective: as a patient. I first noticed how difficult it was to make an appointment and see the doctor when it was convenient for me. Appointments were several weeks or months out and at the most inconvenient times.

Purpose

The purpose of this study is to illuminate patterns of social interaction that influence the behaviors of medical personnel. I also explore how medical personnel interact with patients across race, class, and gender dimensions and try to survive in a cultural situation that can sometimes be hostile. I will utilize the concept of intersectionality to examine the dimensions of medical practitioners in a Midwestern urban hospital setting. Ethnography is the process of choosing between a set of conceptual alternatives and making value-laden judgments to challenge current research on human behavior (Thomas, 1993). Ethnography is a useful hermeneutic approach that does not overly rely on quantitative assessment.

It was clear to me the moment I considered a project and began to learn how to incorporate critical approaches with qualitative methodology; I felt I had an appropriate design to complete my task. Although ethnographers draw their data from direct observations in fieldwork in which the researcher is immersed in another culture, critical researchers attempt to give an emancipatory voice to the subject to empower them or to offer an alternative to a current situation (Thomas, 1993). This methodology is appropriate to my work because it would involve my immersion in the local culture. Secondly, because I had been a member of organizations similar to this particular healthcare institution I had insight on certain cultural norms. This methodology would allow me to record my observations accurately, together with the meanings and perceptions of the participants.

Autoethnography Research

In the last decade, autoethnography has become increasingly popular for scholars across the disciplines of education and communication studies to utilize and consider in pursuing research and pedagogy (Denzin, 2003; Hughes, 2008). According to (White & Seibold, 2008) the term *autoethnography* was first used in the late 1970s by David Hayno in the context of cultural studies conducted by anthropologists to understand the culture of their own population. The research of narrative autoethnography involves the experiences of the ethnographer and analysis of other experiences, with emphasis on the dialogue between the group participants and the narrator (White & Seibold, 2008). According to Hughes (2008), autoethnography research was initially established as a confluence of autoenthnography, theory, pedagogy, and performance ethnography in the groundbreaking work done by Denzin (2003) in his *Performance Ethnography: Critical Pedagogy and the Politics of Culture*. Previous autoethnographic research indicates at least three links to communications studies and autoethnography linked to reflexivity, learning, and teaching (Hughes, 2008).

Goals for this study include the utilization of critical autoethnography, informed by a Black feminist paradigm. Critical ethnography is a type of research embedded in conventional ethnography (Cresswell, 1994). Critical autoethnographic inquiry is being utilized in this project because it provides the best tools for collecting and analyzing data in the setting being studied. For example, people's daily lived experiences cannot be relayed through quantitative methodology. A critical autoethnographic approach begins with the ontological premise that cultural structure and content make life more pleasant. To ensure accuracy in the project, I utilized a triangulation method (Denzin, 1970). Triangulation is a concept that utilizes a combination of methodologies to study the same research setting or question.

The qualitative methods used in this study are autoethnography, oral histories, and interviews. These methods were chosen for two reasons. First, autoethnography enabled me to draw upon my memory, as a member of the medical profession. Second, oral histories and interviews afforded me the chance to collect detailed information about the setting, social interactions, and friendships from informants, which could be used to compare with observations and assumptions formed during the course of this study.

Third, within the context of oral history, the reflections collected can be connected within the larger context of history; for example, Portelli (1997) notes that "we can see how each individual text negotiates the interplay of the personal and the social, of individual expression and social praxis. This negotiation varies with each text and each performance" (p. 82). Therefore, triangulation of autoethnography, oral histories, and interviews are complementary to one another and provide data that can only be assessed through qualitative methodology. Finally, I will utilize a Black feminist critique to draw conclusions from my findings. The basic assumption underlying the Black feminist perspective is that within a contemporary context, collaborative techniques outweigh competitive or confrontational means to solve problems. Therefore, what follows is an account of how my experience became a catalyst for a transformation. My experience also helps to birth a much needed voice for an alternative perspective in healthcare that takes into account the social experiences and beliefs of people of color.

The Complexity of Provider Patient Power Relations

Outpatient care has its own set of issues but inpatient care adds another dimension of dysfunction. I was also able to be an integral part of this system in the fall of 2011. In September 2011, I transitioned from private practice to full-time employment with a local university. The stress of closing my practice, the meetings with lawyers and my new employers caused my lupus to rage out of control. I started developing small, painful ulcerations in my mouth and throat to the point that it became increasingly more difficult to eat or even swallow liquids. I slowly began to lose weight and had little energy or endurance. I continued to work until it was painfully obvious that I was too dehydrated to continue. At this point, because I knew it would almost be impossible to get an appointment with my specialist on such short notice, I contacted my primary care physician (PCP). I warned my doctor that I would need to be admitted to the hospital because on the day I saw her, I was febrile, had lost a significant amount of weight, and looked pretty ill.

My doctor immediately admitted me to one of the local hospitals, and so my new journey began. This first week of my hospitalization educated me on hospital care from the patient's perspective. I always viewed hospitals as places of healing but soon learned that they are the antithesis of healing. Healing cannot occur when patients are sleep deprived, fearful, stressed, and overwhelmed. Although this first group of doctors and nurses were caring, empathetic, and respectful, the hospital stay was still plagued with frequent laboratory tests and interruptions, noisy sleeping conditions, and difficulty getting bathroom assistance when needed. Nurses and care technicians are overworked: they have too many patients.

My experience there would be considered royal as compared to the next experience. Unfortunately, upon discharge from the hospital my health declined. I began having severe flank pain which I assumed came from a kidney stone. within a few days of my initial discharge, due to some alarming indications that the lupus might be damaging my kidneys, I was scheduled to see a kidney specialist. When I arrived for that visit, my pain was so severe, and again I looked so ill, that the kidney specialist decided to admit me to his large teaching hospital. I was none too pleased with his recommendation because my patients had often told me of their unfavorable experiences at this particular hospital, but at this point I had no choice.

I was taken to the admitting and registration department. When patients are severely ill, that process is agonizing. Upon completion of that process, I had to sit in my wheelchair in a waiting area until the transporter arrived to take me to my room. At this point, my pain was so excruciating that the other patients started asking about when my transportation would come. My pain was just that obvious. The wait was so long that the registration clerk herself decided to transport me.

Once I arrived in my room, I was told to wait until the nurse could come and check me in. This is also a time-consuming process. I needed to be given a gown and to have an IV placed in my arm, and I was then asked myriad appropriate questions to start my hospital stay. My pain at this point was 15/10. I begged the nurse to call the doctor immediately. I needed something: Tylenol, ibuprofen, anything. The intern finally arrived, took my history, examined me, and prescribed what he thought was appropriate for my degree of pain. Astoundingly, approximately 4 to 5 hours had elapsed from the time I originally saw the specialist to the time I received medication for my pain. It reduced the level of pain from 15/10 to 10/10.

The medicine the intern prescribed was short acting and was written as needed; that is, I received the medicine only when I asked for it. In a hospital setting, narcotics are not kept on the nursing floors. So when the pain started, I had to push my call light and ask for my nurse. A full 10 minutes later she would come to my room and assess that I was in pain. She would then have to enter that information into the computer and order the medication. The medication would then have to be sent up from the pharmacy. Therefore, 30 minutes or so after I complained of the pain, I would receive some type of relief.

This process went on for days. This particular hospital was situated in an urban environment, often took care of the most indigent individuals in the city, and frequently had to care for persons who simply were seeking drugs. So here I was, a physician with no prior record that I was a drug abuser, my rheumatologist was on staff at the hospital (therefore, my records were easily available for review), and my vital signs indicated that I was indeed in pain: my heart rate was in the 100s, I was breathing fast, and I looked distressed. However, I was treated as if I were seeking drugs. I asked the intern if he would simply prescribe a patient-controlled method of pain (PCA), so that we could stay ahead of the pain. The intern stated that PCAs were only for patients with cancer pain in hospice. That information was incorrect, but that is what he relayed to me.

I was finally able to convince the team that my pain was real, and so I was at last given a PCA. The travesty of my stay continued as the team tried to figure out what was wrong with me. I told them multiple times that I was not taking deep breaths due to the pain. I kept saying to them that something bad was going to happen because of that. When sick patients who are lying in bed for days don't fully inspire and expire, they are at risk of developing pneumonias.

A few days after my admission to this facility, I crashed. I woke up in a panic and could not catch my breath. I could not find the call light, and I barely had enough air in my lungs to scream for help. Fortunately, the door to my room was open and someone walking by heard my cry and got help immediately. My oxygen levels were dropping, and I was crashing. At this point, about 15 people were called to my room and resuscitation began. I was placed on a mask for oxygen, and I was transferred to the Intensive Care Unit (ICU). I knew at that point that I would have to be intubated: placed on a breathing machine.

Because I had just come from a hospitalization for ulcerations in my throat and esophagus, I asked the attending to not allow a resident to intubate me. A resident in the back of the group sarcastically replied: "This *is* a teaching hospital!" As sick as I was at that point, I could not believe what he had just said. I was even more appalled that he had the audacity to say that in front of the attending. I could not imagine a physician in training being that disrespectful to any patient. If he spoke that way to a colleague, imagine how he spoke to those patients far less educated than I.

Before I was actually intubated, I reminded the ICU team that they needed to call my husband and apprise him of my condition. My husband was told that I was not doing well and that I was being transferred to the ICU. Needless to say, that caused him and the rest of my family much anxiety, especially since they thought I had seemed fine the night before. The history of this hospitalization for two days following my intubation was given to me from family and friends, for I have no memory whatever of those days. I was heavily sedated and would go in and out of sleep. Because I was a highly regarded physician in the community, many colleagues came to the hospital as soon as they heard I was ill. Therefore, my husband had some personal friends from whom he could get more information regarding my condition. Just before my mother and my husband walked into my ICU room, a physician friend of ours explained what they would see; he was well aware of how viewing a loved one connected to tubes in every orifice, not breathing on her own, and not being alert, could affect them. The information shared by my friend and not necessarily the hospital staff provided much needed support to my family. You would expect this type of personal care to be a common procedure for staff but unfortunately it does not routinely occur.

At this point, my family was very skeptical about my care. Every detail of my care needed to be explained to them, and they cross-referenced the information with other healthcare professionals whom they trusted. They were also terrified to leave my side. They watched my vitals on the monitor and would become increasingly alarmed if my temperature or heart rate would rise. Having been on the other side of this situation in the past, I am convinced the nursing staff was annoyed. Now that I have experienced this situation as a patient, I see now how healthcare professionals perpetuate their own annoyance by not adequately communicating with the family and providing emotional support. To healthcare staff, this is just a routine day; to that particular family, this is their worst nightmare and they fear the worst.

ICU care can be compared to a highly technical transit system, with the engineers analogous to the nurses and doctors. This system also includes technicians, engineer assistants, maintenance staff, and housekeeping. Just as occurs in a transit system, people are constantly entering and leaving the system. However, the difference in healthcare is that leaving the system could be permanent, as in death. The two systems are also alike in the decibel of their noise. Unless one is sedated, sleeping in a hospital is rare due to the noise, pain, and constant blood draws, X-rays, and interruptions by the healthcare teams.

Although my care was technically excellent, at times the compassion ratio was very low. In the medical workers' defense, ICU shifts are long and hard. Many of the nurses may be caring for two severely ill patients at the same time. These patients are on multiple medications, they need to be cleaned, their IVs are constantly beeping, and their respiratory status could change suddenly. These patients could crash in a moment's notice. The enormous pressure these nurses must face is overwhelming. At the same time, the mental and physical well-being of the patient must be the singular focus. Besides compassion, maintaining the patient's dignity is paramount for a successful hospital experience. My hospital experience definitely took a toll on my self-esteem and pride. I transformed from an extremely independent woman to one who was dependent upon others for basic needs such as toileting and simply rolling from side to side. I recall an instance where the nurses had to clean my entire body due to leakage of my rectal tube. In addition to enduring the look of horror on one of the nurses' faces, I had a male physician walk in on me during this compromising position.

The ultimate indignity I experienced involved my complaints of pain. By the time I was admitted to the ICU, I had been in the hospital for a full two weeks. Even prior to the hospitalization, I had not been eating well for weeks; Therefore, I was extremely weak and I hurt all over. Each day that the team would visit me, I complained of pain, and most places they touched were tender. On the day before I was discharged from the ICU, I overheard them discussing my case and describing me as a drug seeker. I overheard the attending say to the team: "Well, you know how we treat those people." I could not believe that they actually thought that I was seeking narcotics for abuse. Did they come to this conclusion because I was African American? At this point in my care, all I wanted to do was go home. As a physician, medically I understood that I was in no condition to leave the facility. But no human being should endure such horrific indignities. I was so infuriated that my respiratory rate and heart rate were constantly elevated. I could not relax in such a place where I was disrespected and humiliated.

Eventually, I was discharged from intensive care and moved to a regular hospital floor. I was actually placed on a floor where the nursing supervisor was a former patient. She was made aware of my previous experiences and did everything in her power to make the remainder of my stay pleasant. I was so debilitated at this point that the entire treatment team felt I would need inpatient rehabilitation. I was determined to go home, however. Stunned and disgusted by my hospital experience, I was determined to work harder to improve my strength and prove to the physical and occupational therapist that I would do well at home. I relied on my own personal faith for that inner strength to succeed.

I was relieved that my posthospital experience was far more pleasant than the nightmare I had just survived. I was assigned to a phenomenal physical therapist who made me feel human again. She treated me with respect, encouraged me, and pushed my body to its full potential. She also helped restore some of my faith in the healthcare system.

Discussion and Conclusion

Since slavery, Black women have endured horrible indignities. Medical scholar Harriet Washington in her book *Medical Apartheid: The Dark History of Medical Experimentation on Black Americans from Colonial Times to Present* (2004) recounts an example of a female slave who was operated on multiple times without anesthesia by a doctor who is now revered as the father of obstetrics and gynecology. Slave women could be used in any type of experimentation with the consent of the slave master. During the 1800s, women who delivered at home by a midwife often did better medically than those who had to go to a hospital. Previously, it was common practice for doctors to come directly from the morgues to the hospital to see patients. With sterilization and proper hand hygiene an uncommon practice, women who went to the hospital often died of sepsis following delivery. Therefore, the fear of hospital care began. Correspondingly, contemporary health care disparities are strongly related to power relations in the social hierarchy of the medical field and are strongly related to biases of race, gender, and class.

The main assumption of the study that patients who belong to groups that are most frequently represented in disparity studies probably have higher incidences of suffering was correlated. The study contributes to the growing body of literature of power relations and healthcare, which suggests that the understanding, and management of suffering by heath providers is correlated to dimensions of race, gender, and class. The study has the potential to influence the training and clinical practice of healthcare providers by providing a personal account of the patients' own words of the reality of the feelings of suffering and disempowerment during treatment. In conclusion, the study demonstrates and functions as a plea for healthcare providers to develop a greater understanding of the patient's needs in a larger context. The most important implication of this study for healthcare providers and clinical practice is that they promote an approach to healthcare that is sensitive to race, gender, and class.

References

Carlsen, F., & Kaarboe, O. (2010). Norwegian priority guidelines: Estimating the distributional implications across age, gender and SES. *Health Policy, 95*(2–3), 264–270.

Clarke J. N., & James S. (2003). The radicalized self: The impact on the self of the contested nature of the diagnosis of chronic fatigue syndrome. *Social Science and Medicine, 57*, 1387–1395.

Creswell, J. (1994). *Research design: Qualitative and quantitative approaches.* Thousand Oaks, CA: Sage.

De los Reyes, Paulina & Mulinari, Diana (2005) *Intersektionalitet: kritiskareflektioneröver (o)jämlikhetenslandskap*. Malmö: Liber.

Denzin, Norman K. (1970). *The research act: A theoretical introduction to Sociological methods.* Chicago: Aldine Publishing.

Denzin, N. K. (2003). *Performance ethnography: Critical pedagogy and the politics of culture.* Thousand Oaks, CA. Sage.

Eriksson, K. (2006). *The suffering human being.* Chicago: Nordic Studies Press.

Hughes, S. (2008). Toward "good enough methods" for autoethnography in a graduate education course: Trying to resist the Matrix with another promising Red Pill. *Educational Studies: A Journal of the American Education Studies Association, 43*(2), 125–143.

Malterud, K. (2010). Power inequalities in healthcare-empowerment revisited. *Patient Education and Counseling, 79*(2), 139–140.

Morse J. M. (2001). Toward a praxis theory of suffering. *Advances in Nursing Science, 24*(1), 47–49.

Portelli, A. (1997). *The battle of Valle Guilia: Oral history and the art of dialogue.* Madison: University of Wisconsin Press.

Thomas, J. (1993). *Doing critical ethnography.* Newbury Park, CA: Sage.

Washington, H. (2004). *Medical Apartheid: The dark history of medical experimentation on Black Americans from colonial times to present.* New York: Double Day.

White, S., & Seibold, C. (2008). Walk a mile in my shoes: An auto-ethnographic study. *Contemporary Nurse, 30*, 57–68.

Section II

Breast Cancer, the Silence and the Shame

3 Pink Is for (Survivor) Girls
Late-Stage Breast Cancer, Silence, and Pink Ribbon Culture

Elizabeth M. Davis

The public story of breast cancer is a story of survivors, and their families and friends, wearing pink ribbon pins and pink t-shirts, pumping a fist triumphantly in the air while walking, running, or biking for the cure. These women are usually portrayed in popular culture as young, energetic, and living their lives after treatment for an early-stage cancer that has been successfully treated (Carter, 2003). Admittedly, they have gone through some tough times during treatment and recovery, but they have come out whole and ready to get on with life. These women advocate for breast cancer awareness whenever possible, blog their stories on breast cancer support websites, and willingly share their experiences with newly diagnosed breast cancer "survivors."

The missing story in breast cancer culture is the tale told by women diagnosed with late-stage or metastasized breast cancer. The experience of Dr. Suzanne Hebert, a metastatic cancer patient in a breast cancer support group, tells a different tale:

> [T]he room was filled with women who had early localized cancers. Some had completed chemotherapy years ago; they were "survivors." When one newcomer asked Dr. Hebert for her story, she couldn't bring herself to tell the truth. … "This woman had just been diagnosed," Dr. Hebert said of her support-group encounter, "and *I couldn't bring myself to tell her* 'I have it in my bones, I have it in several parts of my body. My treatment is never going to end.' … I had nothing in common with them. I was what scared them" [Emphasis added]
> (Rabin, 2011, p. D1)

Dr. Hebert's story is told, not by what she says within the group, but by her silence, what she cannot say to frightened and hopeful women with breast cancer. The dominant "survivor" discourse surrounding breast cancer legitimizes a set of experiences, acting as a disciplinary mechanism that encourages conformity to one specific set of practices while silencing the diverse experiences of breast cancer and concealing the social, cultural, and political facets underlying those experiences.[1] This chapter considers the importance of addressing the Third Persona (the absent person) constructed through a rhetoric of silence in cultural narratives of breast cancer.

Black (1970) coined the term *Second Persona* to describe the audience implied or constructed through discourse, and Wander (1984) expanded on Black's concept:

> What is negated through the Second Persona forms the silhouette of a Third Persona—the "it" that is not present, that is objectified in a way the "you" and "I" are not. This being not present may, depending on how it is fashioned, become quite alien. ... But "being negated" includes not only being alienated through language—the "it" that is the summation of all that you and I are told to avoid becoming, but also being negated in history, a being whose presence, though relevant to what is said, is negated through silence. (pp. 209–210)

Thus, breast cancer discourse constructs its own history, one where disease is always manageable for women who engage in early detection practices and where women with late-stage cancer are consigned to marginal rhetorical spaces that serve as unspoken background best left unnoticed. Cloud defines rhetoric of silence as "a discursive pattern in which speakers gesture incompletely toward what cannot be uttered in a context of oppression" (1999, p. 178).

Today's emphasis on cause-marketing, and the perpetuation of a "bright-side" (Ehrenreich, 2001) perspective on breast cancer has led to commodification of the disease and cultural dogma that requires a specific performance of the breast cancer patient as the price of full admission into the club. This dogma is endorsed and perpetuated by popular culture, by medical institutions through educational materials for cancer patients and their families, by the public, and by breast cancer advocacy groups.

This chapter is developed in three sections: the development of the dominant and secondary narratives in breast cancer discourses; the impact of pink ribbon culture and the use of *survivor* as an organizing trope in pink ribbon culture; and the uses and strategies of silence within pink ribbon culture.

Breast Cancer Narratives

The two earliest and most important producers of breast cancer literature, the American Cancer Society (ACS) and the National Cancer Institutes (NCI), have a long history and have provided a foundation for current breast cancer discourses (Leopold, 1999; Patterson, 1987). According to Leopold, "[t]he story of breast cancer in the twentieth century is as much about the assimilation of women into the establishment culture as it is about the pace of medical progress" (1999, p. 12). Analysis of patient materials produced by the ACS and NCI reveals two narratives: a dominant, early-stage breast cancer story and a secondary, late-stage breast cancer story (Davis, 1998; 2008). These narratives are distributed across a range of patient support materials and provide a prescription for "good patient" behavior and attitude on the part of women with breast cancer.

"All women are at risk for breast cancer" is a dominant theme in the early-stage narrative. Risk motivates women to participate in early detection practices, helps doctors determine treatment options, and dictates women's behaviors after treatment to minimize the possibility of a recurrent breast cancer. In the primary narrative, the typical breast cancer patient/survivor is a well-informed, proactive, and motivated woman—subtly portrayed as White, middle class, and heterosexual—who attends to her breast health through regular self-examination and mammograms. When she is diagnosed, the breast cancer is always "early stage"; the woman experiences and controls her fear, goes through recommended treatments with manageable discomfort, and utilizes her intellect and strong work ethic to fight the disease on every front. She may become temporarily overwhelmed by a range of normal emotional responses, but these do not permanently incapacitate her. The narrative constructs the experience of breast cancer as individual and reflective of a capitalist work ethic. Problems arise because of actions or conditions unique to the individual, and the success or failure of the outcomes is equally attributable to the diligence and hard work of the individual woman.

Treatment may be temporarily inconvenient but does not cause a permanent change in lifestyle; nor does it seriously limit the woman's ability to return to her life as a productive worker. Yet, cancer is also transformative. Danger and opportunity combined, cancer changes what this woman values, brings new insights, and leads to closer intimacy with her loved ones. Cancer catalyzes positive change while leaving the woman, in her most significant inner recesses, unmarked by cancer.

In addition to the early-stage narrative that dominates medical discourses, there is a second narrative that tells an advanced cancer story (Davis, 1998). This narrative is isolated to a select few support materials in the ACS and NCI literature and reflects the marginalization of women with late-stage breast cancer, which is framed as terminal. Risk is irrelevant for the terminal patient. Future illness is no longer a concern, and uncertainty has vanished. Advanced breast cancer establishes a dying trajectory for the patient and, in its nature as terminal, creates an air of hopelessness. However, the advanced cancer narrative adds both a holistic aspect and a spiritual dimension to its definition of health and illness. In this story, a woman is diagnosed with advanced cancer, either late-stage or metastatic. The same cultural and class assumptions apply to the late-stage cancer patient. If this is recurrent cancer, the woman is temporarily suspended between the primary and secondary narratives until her doctor determines that her cancer is truly "advanced," thus plunging the woman into the late-stage cancer story. She knows she is dying, yet she is challenged by cancer and will not give up in despair. In this story the woman with late-stage breast cancer often becomes more interested in spiritual or religious issues and engages in prayer or meditation. Over the course of the narrative, the woman experiences the classic five stages of grief: denial, anger, bargaining, depression, and finally, acceptance (Kubler-Ross, 1969).

The narratives found in medical discourse are reproduced in other breast cancer discourses. Patient advocacy services such as Reach to Recovery, popular culture references and storylines in television programs such as *Murphy Brown* and *Sex and the City*, and advice columns and articles on breast health, all offer the same basic story of successful treatment, wholeness of appearance, and recovery of one's life as it was before cancer. Survivor blogs and breast cancer support groups also participate in this regime of practices, allowing women with breast cancer to offer support and suggestions, and answer questions for other women with breast cancer. Bloggers and support group members serve to police attitudes and behaviors by admonishing women for negative attitudes and redirecting focus toward the survivor storyline (Ehrenreich, 2001). The late-stage narrative is explicitly told in isolated texts but is implied in the interstices of the early-stage story. When women are told that mammograms can save lives and find breast cancer at the earliest possible stages, the consequences of not finding cancer early resonate in the silence. What is not told outright becomes the thing to fear and avoid.

Although the public discourses of breast cancer focus on individual agency, understanding cultural narrative is vital to empowering both individual choice and collective action. According to Fisher (1987), people are "authors and co-authors who creatively read and evaluate the texts of life and literature" (p. 18). Narrative "gives prominence to human agency and imagination" (Riessman, 1993, p. 5), facilitating better understanding of the ways in which cultural narratives enable and constrain the articulation of human values through discourse (Fisher, 1987).

Pink Ribbon Culture and Its Narrative Construction

Pink ribbon culture is marked by several features that appeal to a mass audience but that deeply disturb many breast cancer activists and critical scholars. The public image of breast cancer carefully cultivated by many mainstream breast cancer groups reinforces and is reinforced by the early-stage cancer narrative endorsed in medical discourses and epitomized by the survivor metaphor. The cause-marketing that turns October into a pink nightmare for many women with cancer leads to an endless array of pink products and corporate-sponsored events that force women with breast cancer to become hyper-aware of their cancer status (King, 2006).

According to Bartels (2009), the term *survivor* first appeared in 1985 in "unassuming 'occasional notes'" in the *New England Journal of Medicine*, which "would become the starting point for a major medical and cultural shift in the United States, ... a revolutionary change in focus from cancer patients to cancer 'survivors'" (p. 237). The term was not used originally to refer to women with breast cancer, but was quickly adopted within the breast cancer community and "was used strategically to destigmatize the disease and to empower women to take personal and collective action" (Sulik, 2011, p. 34). King (2006) labels pink ribbon culture one of "survivorship" where a "tyranny of cheerfulness" dominates (p. 101). Survivors in pink ribbon culture "are uniformly youthful (if not always young), ultrafeminine, slim, immaculately groomed, radiant with health, joyful, and seemingly at peace with the world" (King, 2006, p. 102). This ideal of femininity is reflected in images used in association with breast cancer and in beauty practices advocated by breast cancer organizations to help women "look normal" after cancer.

Ucok (2007) supports this conclusion of extreme femininity in her analysis of institutionalized representations of women with breast cancer through the "Look Good, Feel Better" program offered by the ACS. She notes that the use of before and after images participates in "a dominant cultural discourse on *gendered appearance* [that] provide a model for the reader regarding what is 'acceptable' and 'beautiful'" (p. 71). Ucok (2007) compared these traditional models with visual images that create "alternative discourses," offering an expansion of conventional definitions of beauty (pp. 74–75). These alternate images depict women with mastectomy scars—unadorned or tattooed, bald heads without the camouflage of wigs, bodies marked by disease and displayed without shame or fear. Such images refute the pseudo-wholeness so carefully constructed in mainstream representations of breast cancer survivors (Young, 1992).

Reassurance for women with breast cancer comes in the form of clothing and makeup to mask signs of illness or defect, soothing tokens, and pink products of every imaginable kind. Corporations have found a fruitful avenue for marketing in the public discourse of breast cancer. Perpetuating the myth of an ideal womanhood, product manufacturers participate in a cancer-industrial complex whose interests are served by maintaining a narrative of personal control and feminine beauty that "positions them as pro-women but not feminist. This model also helps to maintain support for high-stakes, early detection, and cure-oriented research to the virtual exclusion of other avenues of exploration" (King, 2006, p. 104). Commodification of breast cancer demands this focus on early-stage disease and the culture of survivorship; terminal patients are less likely to shop, whereas survivors have greater incentive to "celebrate life" and reward themselves through consumption of goods and services. Ehrenreich (2001) questions whether

> [c]ulture' is too weak a word to describe all this. What has grown up around breast cancer in just the last fifteen years more nearly resembles a cult—or, given that it numbers more than two million women, their families, and friends—perhaps we should say a full-fledged religion. The products—teddy bears, pink-ribbon brooches, and so forth—serve as amulets and talismans, comforting the sufferer and providing visible evidence of faith. (p. 50)

This fervor is evident in contemporary discourse where early detection equals prevention; mammography becomes a shield against disease, even though that shield is both false and, potentially, a contributor to the very disease it seeks to find. Controversy over the efficacy of annual mammography before age 50, both in terms of detection and exposure to radiation, led to a revision of medical guidelines for early detection practices. So well-entrenched is the pink ribbon cultural narrative that women were outraged that one of their "lifelines" to "prevention" would be curtailed (Ehrenreich, December 9, 2009).

The survivor metaphor so boldly advocated in pink ribbon culture provides a single labeling practice within which to construct personal meaning. Survivors are fighters, warriors who have beaten the odds and defeated an enemy, or at least who have taken the worst the enemy had to give and lived through the ordeal to fight another day. This trope "was made visible through such figures as Betty Ford, Shirley Temple Black, and Happy Rockefeller, icons of all-American, hypernormal femininity" (King, 2006, p. 112). Many women wholeheartedly embrace this metaphor, for the very reason that it confers status as a finisher and a winner. But others are either uncomfortable with the label or reject it outright.

> For those who cease to be survivors and join the more than 40,000 American women who succumb to breast cancer each year—again, no noun applies. They are said to have "lost their battle" and may be memorialized by photographs carried at races for the cure–our lost, brave sisters, our fallen soldiers. But in the overwhelmingly Darwinian culture that has grown up around breast cancer, martyrs count for little; it is the "survivors" who merit constant honor and acclaim. They, after all, offer living proof that expensive and painful treatments may in some cases actually work.
>
> (Ehrenreich, 2001, p. 48)

The desperate need of women with breast cancer to believe that these painful and often debilitating treatments to which they willingly submit will repatriate them into the country of the healthy leads to a shunning of women with metastatic or late-stage breast cancer. "Survivors" do not participate in a rhetoric of failure. The metaphor of survivorship depends on submission to science and medicine (King, 2006). The late-stage breast cancer narrative focuses on the failure of medicine and so must be silenced whenever possible.

The sick role described by Parsons and others (Brody, 1987; Kleinman, 1988) is redeemed in pink ribbon culture through the use of restitution and quest narratives (Frank, 1995), both individually and in the cultural narrative of survivorship. Restitution narratives are a general story type characterized by the themes of health, sickness, and a return to health (Frank, 1995). Quest narratives, another story type, are characterized by the theme of illness as a challenge or journey that requires departure, initiation, and return—"no longer ill, but remain[ing] marked by illness" in a transformative fashion (Frank, 2006, p. 118). The late-stage cancer narrative found in institutionalized discourse reinforces these concepts of restitution and quest through silence and the act of failure. If sickness leads to recovery and normalcy, perhaps even new insights, then those who are "terminally ill" reside beyond the sick role, in a place that survivors need not contemplate.

Similarly, through the normalizing discourse of pink ribbon culture, all women share the potential experience of breast cancer, thereby eliminating the stigma once so strongly associated with the disease. In contrast, because it represents failure, the late-stage cancer narrative takes up the full mantle of stigmatization. Metastatic or late-stage breast cancer becomes publicly shameful in the same way any breast cancer diagnosis was once shameful.

Pink ribbon culture denies the political dimension of breast cancer, effectively obliterating the link between micro and macro processes. Women who identify with pink ribbon culture willingly or unconsciously relinquish awareness of political conditions associated with breast cancer and the power of political protest as a means of rectification. The late-stage breast cancer narrative reinforces this position by reminding women of the losses they face should they slip into this narrative realm. The *survivor* metaphor serves to frame the cult of individual responsibility—the pink ribbon culture narrative makes "survivorship" and "success" a personal quest and responsibility. If women don't get better, it must be because they didn't try hard enough. This position is held in tension with the overt claims that late-stage patients are not blamed for their cancers or for not "winning the war" against breast cancer.

Strategies of Silence in Pink Ribbon Culture

At the beginning of his book on "silence and denial in everyday life," Zerubavel (2006) recounts an early version of the fable known as "The Emperor's New Clothes," in which a royal ruler is tricked into believing that three weavers have created a stunning new robe for him to wear (pp. 1–3). The "trick" is that the cloth is invisible to anyone not of legitimate birth. Because no one wants to be accused of being illegitimate, all of the ruler's advisors declare the new robe a masterpiece. The ruler, wanting to retain credibility with his people, marvels at the elegant new clothing. He parades through the city wearing his invisible new robe, and none among his subjects will dare to point out the obvious—that the King isn't wearing any clothes. No one is willing to look foolish or be shunned as illegitimate, until one man, a servant without much to lose, finally calls out "the King is naked."

The moral of this story, that few will speak when there is risk of public censure, is explained in part by the spiral of silence theory, which argues that silence is motivated by fear of isolation in the public sphere (Noelle-Neumann, 1993). Noelle-Neumann (1993) theorizes that people shape their opinions based on what they perceive to be the majority public opinion on a given issue, and fear of isolation will compel people to remain silent if they perceive that their perspective does not match the majority public opinion.

Scheufele (2008) describes the spiral of silence as a dynamic process that develops over time: "As people who perceive themselves to be in the minority fall silent, perceptions of opinion climates shift over time, and ultimately the majority opinion is established as the predominant one or even as a social norm" (pp. 4–5). Further, Scheufele identifies "two contingent conditions" that impact the spiraling process: a moral component, and media attention to the issue (p. 5). Gonzenbach, King, and Jablonski (1999) argue that the spiral of silence is useful particularly when considering subgroups:

> The spiral of silence assumes that an individuals's [sic] opinions and behavior regarding specific issues are influenced by the fear of isolation. ... The lack of effect for perceptions of the majority might be explained by the observation that people are not attempting to conform to an undifferentiated majority. Instead, they may only be concerned about and influenced by certain subgroups.
>
> (Gonzenbach et al., 1999, p. 295)

Their argument supports the idea that the spiral of silence is useful in terms of its underlying assumptions, not public opinion per se; and in the case of pink ribbon culture, the influence of certain subgroups and "publics" might be more relevant to understanding narrative discourses and strategies of silence in managing the dominant narrative.

As a "reaction to openly visible approval and disapproval among shifting constellations of values" (Noelle-Neumann, 1993, p. 64), the spiral of silence facilitates a better understanding of how strategies of silencing are used to maintain an upbeat and cheerful focus on survivorship within pink ribbon culture. There are three meanings of public in this theory: the legal sense (e.g., public places, spaces, and events); the rights and force sense (e.g., state involvement, public interests, and "the general welfare"); and the sociopsychological sense (e.g., those pressures and conditions, unrelated to legal/place concepts or state control, that shape individual and collective behaviors, thoughts, and practices) (Noelle-Neumann, 1993, p. 61). The trope of survivorship relies on the third meaning, the sociopsychological, or what Noelle-Neumann (1993) also calls our "social skin": that set of normative behaviors and practices that enable and constrain participants in pink ribbon culture.

Research on breast cancer narratives and the first-person stories of women with breast cancer suggest three broad categories of silencing strategy: passive and active silencing, which includes practices of denial, avoidance, absence, and invisibility; stigmatizing and shaming; and practices of consumption and commodification.

Active and Passive Silencing

Silence, including denial, avoidance, absence, and invisibility, is used in pink ribbon culture discourses both passively and actively. Women are introduced into pink ribbon culture through a specific early-stage cancer story and a particular set of labels, images, and practices. Just as when they were newly arrived in the world and wrapped in a pink blanket and cap to identify them as legitimate members of womankind, women entering the world of breast cancer are given iconic pink talismans and wrapped in pink words and images to identify them as legitimate members of pink ribbon culture. This acculturation acts as a covert means to silence dissenting voices (Clair, 1997). A prescriptive early-stage cancer narrative, survivor and war metaphors, and a perpetual bombardment of pink awareness messages and symbols frame what can and cannot be comfortably spoken in pink ribbon culture. "[W]omen ... [are] silenced in a cacophony of pink talk" (Sulik, 2011, p. 317).

The early-stage narrative limits the entrance point into this discourse. Naming provides a vocabulary and a forum for discourse (Charmaz, 2002). As a strategy for providing voice, naming clearly empowers discourse. As a strategy for silence, cultural narratives of early detection and survivorship name breast cancer in specific terms that offer little room for culturally acceptable alternative stories (Charmaz, 2002; Clair, 1997, 1998). Women who are diagnosed with an advanced-stage breast cancer have no easy entry into the culture—except to deny or avoid their status and participate "as if" they too belong in this story. Their alternatives are to reject the support that comes with participation in the culture (a support that women with breast cancer desperately need and usually want), or to enter the discourse with an opposing narrative that often earns them both subtle and overt censure by other women with breast cancer who have fully embraced the survivor metaphor and pink ribbon cultural narrative (AnnMarie, 2012; Ehrenreich, 2001).

Survivor and war metaphors are troubling for women with breast cancer at both ends of the spectrum (Garrison, 2007; Kaiser, 2008). Those women with late-stage or metastasized cancer almost certainly won't survive; they must choose between not participating in the discourses of pink ribbon culture (an act of active absence) or pretending they will fight so they can feel included without frightening other "survivors" or being actively ostracized (an act of passive denial). Whether through self-exile, self-definition, or denial by silence, they perceive themselves as excluded from the discourse. In interviews with 39 women treated for breast cancer, Kaiser (2008) found that some women preferred the trope of warrior rather than survivor, and others rejected the term *survivor* because they feared recurrent cancer—the survivor metaphor failed to account for their feelings of uncertainty. Yet others rejected the term *survivor* because they were facing chronic or otherwise stigmatizing disease, and they feared that the term would limit their social definition of self to their disease condition. Some women with breast cancer reject the warrior metaphor as a poor expression of their values toward public protest and peace (Garrison, 2007).

Likewise, extreme optimism seems to be a point of difficulty at times in balancing the cheerfulness of pink ribbon culture and the emotions inherent in a breast cancer diagnosis (Coreil, Wilke, & Pintado, 2004; Ehrenreich, 2001; Kitzinger, 2000). Kitzinger (2000) found that women attempted to counteract the oft-heard but vague phrase "think positive" through "production of competing idioms" (an active naming strategy to counteract silence, but one that is likely to re-inscribe cultural norms); "pauses and token agreements" (partial acts of silence); and "particularization" (accepting or refusing conversational affiliation, which can lead to avoidance).

Cultural factors also impact women's perception of breast cancer discourse. Pink ribbon culture, as suggested earlier, is a predominantly White heterosexual, middle-class phenomenon (Davis, 1998, 2004). Research shows that women of color consistently feel silenced by the discourses that surround them after a breast cancer diagnosis (Barnes, 2008; Borrayo, Buki, & Feigal, 2005; hooks, 1993; Jain, 2007; Lende & Lachiondo, 2009; Olson, 1997; Ryan, 2004; Thomas, 2006). Many women of color lament the lack of embodied experience in breast cancer discourses and feel as if pink ribbon culture has little to offer them regarding body image issues in relation to illness (hooks, 1993; Lorde, 1980; Yalom, 1997). Black, lesbian, feminist, author, activist Audre Lorde (1980) articulated the many ways in which the medical system and available breast cancer support resources failed to address her needs as a Black woman, or even seemingly to consider that she might have needs different from those of a White woman. In all of these instances, women of color are made invisible within pink ribbon culture, either through a lack of adequate language through which to express their experiences or through a lack of images to represent them as participating within breast cancer culture.

Similarly, there is a history of lesbians experiencing a variety of biases in relation to illness and medical treatment (Barnes, 2008; Jain, 2007; Olson, 1997). Lesbian women often encounter ostracism, or they choose passive denial of their sexuality as the price of access to the supportive environment of breast cancer culture (Brandt, 1993; Brownworth, 1993; Butler & Rosenblum, 1991; Lorde, 1980, Matthews, Peterman, Delaney, Menard, & Brandenburg, 2002, Rubin & Tanenbaum, 2011). Audre Lorde's experience as a Black lesbian was doubly silencing, and women still report "gender policing" within breast cancer support networks of their choices not to have reconstructive surgeries (Rubin & Tanenbaum, 2011).

Stigmatizing and Shaming

Many women experience shame as a result of pink ribbon discourses, particularly if they have chosen not to engage in reconstructive surgery after a mastectomy or lumpectomy or have other temporary or permanent signs of illness (Bahar, 2003; Bell, 2002; Lorde, 1980; Schultz, 2009). As the visible sign of femininity, breasts are iconic, and the loss or imperfection of a breast signifies more than mere bodily damage (Yalom, 1997; Young, 1992). Bell (2002) analyzes the visual narrative of a photographic project by British feminist Jo Spence from 1982, when she was diagnosed with breast cancer, to 1992, when she died. Spence's photographs have "moral force. 'I Framed My Breast for Posterity' simultaneously reveals and criticizes the ways in which cancer is not spoken about, the ways people with cancer are metaphorically and literally silenced, and how people can search for speech" (Bell, 2002, p. 23). The model Matuschka posed for the cover of *The New York Times Magazine* in 1993 wearing a dress that revealed her mastectomy scar; and in 2011, photographer David Jay created a project online and in book form titled *The Scar Project* to showcase 50 portraits of women under 40 who had been treated for breast cancer. Schultz (2009) analyzes her own embodied experience with breast cancer, chemotherapy, and baldness to better understand the self in relation to bodily experience and appearance and as a way to find new metaphors that reach beyond the victim/victor dichotomy of pink ribbon culture. Such photographic narratives also challenge social science interpretations and stigmatization of illness.

For Jain (2007), the destiny of gender is itself stigmatizing, and she compares the gendered stigma of mastectomy with the successful destigmatization enacted within the HIV/AIDS activist community. Rather than the mantra of HIV/AIDS activism, "silence=death," Jain sees a more appropriate symbol to represent breast cancer: "ubiquity=death" (p. 506). At the other end of the spectrum, Kahane (1990) reported the story of Hemlotta, a woman from India, whose response to her treatment choice for breast cancer was: "I don't want to suffer any stigma that I didn't treat myself properly" (p. 166). Hemlotta was concerned that if her cancer was not cured, she would be blamed for not accepting the correct treatment.

Gray, Sinding, and Fitch (2001) report on the efforts of women with metastatic breast cancer to affirm their own experiences, engage in social action, and resist the stereotypes of pink ribbon culture through theatrical performance. Public performance allowed these women to develop a deeper personal understanding of their lives and educate friends, family, and community members at the same time, but they also had to confront the stigmatizing label of metastatic cancer patient. Projects such as these enact resistance to the standard discourses and imagery of pink ribbon culture, but they also stand as the exceptions that prove the rule. For every woman who feels brave enough to challenge pink ribbon culture and expose her secrets, and often her body, there are thousands more who cannot afford to reject the comfort and support of the dominant cultural narrative.

Practices of Consumption and Commodification

Within pink ribbon culture, as in other aspects of American culture, the mantra for all good citizens, particularly women, is "go shopping." This mantra is proudly and actively upheld in pink ribbon culture, particularly during Breast Cancer Awareness Month. Women become both consumers and commodities within pink ribbon culture; they consume and are consumed for the cause.

"Saving yogurt lids, selecting pink ribbon adorned products, wearing pink bracelets, affixing pink magnetic ribbons to one's car are all examples of everyday activism. While not pivotal in leading to a cure as yet, the increased awareness that comes from these actions undoubtedly leads women to be more diligent about examination and mammography" (Selleck, 2010, p. 135). Selleck argues here that the Susan G. Komen for the Cure Foundation's (SGK) pink marketing creates activists, and she is not alone in her belief (Milden, 2005). However, these conclusions assume that the act of consumption equates action with activism. The statistics shown on the SGK site are not necessarily linked to the organization's practices or to acts of consumption of pink products. The numbers give the appearance of a causal relationship, but appearances can be deceiving. King (2006) notes the "general tendency to deploy consumption as a major avenue of political participation" (p. xxv), thereby diverting effective collective action and reinvesting individual responsibility.

The "cancer-industrial complex" profits from the drug and technology sales associated with breast cancer prevention and treatment (more than they might if a cause and/or actual prevention measures were discovered); and product manufacturers profit from product sales—some related directly to breast cancer, and others simply because of the breast cancer logo slapped on their products. Many organizations and businesses claim to be raising funds for breast cancer awareness and patient advocacy, but when pressed for details and evidence of actual donations, many of these organizations fail to live up to their hype (Goldman, 2011; King, 2006). Ehrenreich (2001) advocates a more direct approach to what she describes as the "relentless brightsiding" in pink ribbon culture (p. 49). She rails against what she sees as a cancer-industrial complex run amok and advocates challenging the assumed truths and practices that keep pink ribbon culture going strong.

Beyond consuming as a measure of their participation in and devotion to pink ribbon culture, breast cancer "survivors," family, and friends become commodities to be consumed by corporations and by the public. Fundraising activities such as the races and walks sponsored by SGK, Avon, and other advocacy groups and corporate sponsors are magnets for corporate "sponsorship" and give-aways of pink ribbon products. The extent and magnitude of this process is well documented (King, 2006; Klawiter, 2008; Sulik, 2011). Women with breast cancer, their families, and their friends become the products marketed to companies as potential consumers—and the circle is complete. Once invested in the cycle of consumption by supporting breast cancer "awareness" through shopping and fundraising, it becomes difficult to see one's actions as anything but productive toward preventing breast cancer or finding a cure. The fact that these practices are not directed in any significant way toward the underlying causes of breast cancer, and so cannot support genuine prevention, is lost in a flurry of seemingly productive practices.

Yet these practices, however, ineffective at producing real progress or change, are not extended to women with late-stage or metastasized breast cancer. These women have little vested interest in practices of consumption and are less likely to spend their way to survivorship in the pink ribbon marketplace. And, by virtue of their stigmatized status, women with late-stage or metastasized breast cancer are not the ideal commodities to "sell" in the pink ribbon marketplace.

Conclusion

In her research, Segal (2008) raises concerns about the very act of narrative that is so prevalent in pink ribbon culture:

> Personal narrative is itself a pink genre; it is so welcome in part because it is unthreatening – unlike, for example, the genre of the protest rally or the diatribe. Furthermore, it is an egocentric genre: it honours the individual and neglects the collective. As long as the personal narrative dominates public discourse on breast cancer, some questions will be suppressed, even silenced, and a degree of ignorance about the disease will be maintained.
>
> (Segal, 2008, p. 17)

Within that silence can be found the Third Persona articulated by Wander (1984). This is the absent audience, the women with late-stage or metastasized breast cancer, the women who find pink teddy bears infantilizing, and the women and men who see collective political action as the means to move forward and find viable solutions to breast cancer.

Segal argues that the very act of questioning the genre of narrative can help to energize the discussion, but she implies that more effective strategies of resistance and change would involve more direct collective action. Ultimately, that action will involve local, regional, and eventually national collectives of women and men who understand and can articulate the power of collective action and who can disrupt the existing regime of practices so that those in the Third Persona can participate in a multivoiced, multifaceted cultural narrative.

Note

1. Foucault uses the term *regimes of practices* to encompass the intersection of discourses, behaviors, social norms and rules, and rationales. Analysis of these practices entails both the "prescriptive effects regarding what is to be done ... and codifying effects regarding what is to be known" (1987, p. 103). Cf. Clair (1998) and Klawiter (2004, 2008).

References

AnnMarie. (2012, June 12). In the midst of silence. [Web log comment]. Retrieved from http://metavivor-blog.com/blog/2012/06/19/in-the-midst-of-silence.

Bahar, S. (2003). "If I'm one of the victims, who survives?": Marilyn Hacker's breast cancer Texts. *Signs, 28,* 1025–1052.

Barnes, S. L. (2008). Marvelous arithmetics: Prosthesis, speech, and death in the late work of Audre Lorde. *Women's Studies, 37,* 769–789.

Bartels, E. C. (2009). Outside the box: Surviving survival. *Literature and Medicine, 28*(2), 237–252.

Bell, S. E. (2002). Photo images: Jo Spence's narratives of living with illness. *Health, 6*(1), 5–30.

Black, E. (1970). The second persona. *Quarterly Journal of Speech, 56*(2), 109–119.

Borrayo, E. A., Buki, L. P., & Feigal, B. M. (2005). Breast cancer detection among older Latinas: Is it worth the risk? *Qualitative Health Research, 15*(9), 1244–1263.

Brandt, Kate. (1993, September–October). Lesbians at risk: Breast cancer. *Deneuve,* 34–37.

Brody, H. (1987). *Stories of sickness.* New Haven, CT: Yale University Press.

Brownworth, Victoria. (1993, February–March). The other epidemic: Lesbians and breast cancer. *Out,* 60–63.

Butler, S., & Rosenblum, B. (1991). *Cancer in two voices.* San Francisco: Spinsters.

Carter, T. (2003). Body count: Autobiography of women living with breast cancer. *Journal of Popular Culture, 36*(4), 653–668.

Charmaz, K. (2002). Stories and silences: Disclosures and self in chronic illness. *Qualitative Inquiry, 8*(3), 302–328.

Clair, R. P. (1997). Organizing silence: Silence as voice and voice as silence in the narrative exploration of the treaty of new Echota. *Western Journal of Communication, 61*(3), 315–337.

Clair, R. P. (1998). *Organizing silence: A world of possibilities.* New York: State University of New York Press.

Cloud, D. L. (1999). The null persona: Race and the rhetoric of silence in the uprising of '34. *Rhetoric and Public Affairs, 2,* 177–209.

Coreil, J. Wilke, J., & Pintado, I. (2004). Cultural models of illness and recovery in breast cancer support groups. *Qualitative Health Research, 14,* 905–923.

Davis, E. M. (1998). From pre-symptomatic to post-recovery and back again: A narrative analysis of medical discourse on breast cancer. (Unpublished doctoral dissertation). The Ohio State University, Columbus, OH.

Davis, E. M. (2008). Risky business: Medical discourse, breast cancer and narrative. *Qualitative Health Research, 18,* 65–76.

Ehrenreich, B. (2001, November). Welcome to cancerland: A mammogram leads to a cult of pink kitsch. *Harper's Magazine, 303*(1818), 43.

Ehrenreich, B. (2009, December 9). Slap on a pink ribbon, call it a day. *Salon.* Retreived from http://www.salon.com/2009/12/02/womens_health_2/#.

Fisher, W. R. (1987). *Human communication as narration: Toward a philosophy of reason, value, and action.* Columbia: University of South Carolina Press.

Foucault, M. (1987). Questions of method: An interview with Michel Foucault. In K. Baynes, J. Bohman, & T. McCarty (Eds.), *After philosophy—end or transformation?* (pp. 100–117). Boston: MIT Press.

Frank, A. W. (1995). *The wounded storyteller: Body, illness, and ethics.* Chicago: University of Chicago Press.

Friedman, D. B. (2010). Breaking the silence: Talking about illness. *Journal of Individual Psychology, 66*(3), 315–322.

Garrison, K. (2007). The personal is rhetorical: War, protest, and peace in breast cancer narratives. *Disability Studies Quarterly, 27*(4). Retrieved from http://dsq-sds.org/issue/view/3.

Goldman, L. (2011, October). The big business of breast cancer. *Marie Claire*, 155–160.

Gonzenbach, W. J., King, C., & Jablonski, P. (1999). Homosexuals and the military: An analysis of the spiral of silence. *The Howard Journal of Communications, 10*, 281–296.

Gray, R. E., Sinding, C., & Fitch, M. I. (2001). Navigating the social context of metastatic breast cancer: Reflections on a project linking research to drama. *Health, 5*, 233–248.

Hall, L., & Donovan, B. (2007). Popular culture representations of breast cancer and their impact on women of different ages. *Conference Papers—American Sociological Association*, 1.

hooks, bell. (1993). *Sisters of the yam: Black women and self-recovery*. Boston: South End.

Jain, S. L. (2007). Cancer butch. *Cultural Anthropology, 22*(4), 502–538.

Kahane, D. H. (1990). *No less a woman: Ten women shatter the myths about breast cancer*. New York: Prentice Hall.

Kaiser, K. (2008). The meaning of survivor identity for women with breast cancer. *Social Science & Medicine, 67*, 79–87.

King, S. (2006). *Pink ribbons, inc.: Breast cancer and the politics of philanthropy*. Minneapolis: University of Minneapolis Press.

Kitzinger, C. (2000). How to resist an idiom. *Research on language and social interaction, 33*(2), 121–154.

Klawiter, M. (2004). Breast cancer in two regimes: The impact of social movements on illness experience. *Sociology of Health and Illness, 26*, 845–874.

Klawiter, M. (2008). The biopolitics of breast cancer: Changing cultures of disease and activism. Minneapolis: University of Minnesota Press.

Kleinman, A. (1988). *The illness narratives: Suffering, healing and the human condition*. New York: Basic.

Kubler-Ross, E. (1969). *On death and dying*. New York: Macmillan.

Lende, D. H., & Lachiondo, A. (2009). Embodiment and breast cancer among African American women. *Qualitative Health Research, 19*(2), 216–228.

Leopold, E. (1999). *A darker ribbon: Breast cancer, women, and their doctors in the twentieth century*. Boston: Beacon.

Lorde, A. (1980). *The cancer journals*. San Francisco: Spinsters.

Matthews, A. K., Peterman, A. H., Delaney, P., Menard, L., & Brandenburg, D. (2002). A Qualitative exploration of the experiences of lesbian and heterosexual patients with breast cancer. *Oncology Nursing Forum, 29*(10), 1455–1462.

Milden, R. (2005). Pink ribbons and bad girls of breast cancer. *Psychoanalysis, Culture and Society, 10*, 98–104.

Noelle-Neumann, E. (1993). *The spiral of silence: public opinion—our social skin* (2nd ed.). Chicago: University of Chicago.

Olson, L. C. (1997). On the margins of rhetoric: Audre Lorde transforming silence into language and action. *Quarterly Journal of Speech, 83*(1), 49–70.

Patterson, James T. (1987). *The dread disease: Cancer and modern American culture*. Cambridge, MA: Harvard University Press.

Rabin, R. C. (2011, January 18). A pink-ribbon race, years long. *The New York Times*, p. D1.

Riessman, C. K. *Narrative analysis*. Newbury Park, CA: Sage, 1993.

Rubin, L. R., & Tanenbaum, M. (2011). "Does that make me a woman?": Breast cancer, mastectomy, and breast reconstruction decisions among sexual minority women. *Psychology of Women Quarterly, 35*(3), 401–414.

Ryan, C. (2004). "Am I not a woman?" The rhetoric of breast cancer stories in African American women's popular periodicals. *Journal of Medical Humanities, 25*(2), 129–150.

Scheufele, D. A. (2008). 16 Spiral of silence theory. In W. Donsback & M. W. Traugott (Eds.), *The SAGE handbook of public opinion research*. (pp.175–184). DOI: 10.4135/9781848607910.n17.

Schultz, J. E. (2009). (Un)body double: A rhapsody on hairless identity. *Literature and Medicine, 28*(2), 371–393.

Segal, J. Z. (2007). Breast cancer narratives as public rhetoric genre itself and the maintenance of ignorance. *Linguistics and the Human Sciences, 3*(1), 3–23.

Selleck, L. G. (2010). Pretty in pink: The Susan G. Komen network and the branding of the breast cancer cause. *Nordic Journal of English Studies, 9*(3), 119–138.

Sulik, G. A. (2011). Pink ribbon blues: How breast cancer culture undermines women's health. New York: Oxford University Press.

Thomas, E. (2006). Ring of silence: African American women's experiences related to their breasts and breast cancer screening. *The Qualitative Report, 2*(11), 350–373.

Ucok, O. (2007). The fashioned survivor: Institutionalized representations of women with breast cancer. *Communication and Medicine, 4*(1), 67–78.

Wander, P. (1984). The third persona: An ideological turn in rhetorical theory. *Central States Speech Journal, 35*, 197–216.

Yalom, M. (1997). *A history of the breast*. New York: Alfred A. Knopf.

Young, I. M. (1992). Breasted experience: The look and the feeling. In Leder, D. (Ed.), *The body in medical thought and practice* (pp. 215–230). Dordrecht, The Netherlands: Kluwer Academic Press.

Zerubavel, E. (2006). *The elephant in the room: Silence and denial in everyday life*. New York: Oxford University Press.

4 Breast Cancer and Shame

Problematizing the Pink Ribbon in Locations of Women's Breast Healthcare

Sarah Hochstetler

A few months ago I had a routine mammogram at a women's health center in a midsized Midwestern city. Between changing out of my blouse and bra and being called back into the imaging area, I sat in the communal patient suite with three other smocked women. In the spirit of Barbara Ehrenreich's (2001) analysis and evaluation of the mammogram as a site for induction into the world of breast cancer, I performed a cursory inventory of the room's contents and observed other patients. I took note of the following: one woman picking up and reading a well-worn copy of *Chicken Soup for the Breast Cancer Survivor's Soul* (2006); another investigating the varied posters on the walls serving to advertise an upcoming Avon "Walk for Breast Cancer"; and a third flipping through an album of images of office employees at previous years' local Komen "Race for the Cure" walks and runs. This space also contained a sampling of other ultrafeminized pink or pink-ribboned objects related to the prevention of breast cancer, in-treatment cancer support, and life after the disease. Taken in whole, these artifacts send patients a clear message: The pink ribbon movement and the values it espouses is the preferred framework for understanding and engaging breast cancer in this location.

During my research about the rhetoric of breast cancer, I have visited many medical spaces where women seek consultations about or therapy for breast cancer, including offices for reproductive health and chemotherapy infusion rooms. The vast majority of these sites prominently displayed support of the pink ribbon movement. Such sites paraded informative pamphlets, posters, and other materials promoting the pink ribbon movement. Few would be surprised to see the ubiquitous pink ribbon in a venue for breast health, especially in the Komen-saturated years following Ehrenreich's (2001) critique of what she describes as the breast cancer cult. But what goes unanalyzed in this intrusion of pink is the ways the values inherent in the pink ribbon movement infiltrate these spaces as well, and how practitioners, by displaying their "support," are also sanctioning a specific framework for breast cancer that can serve to discipline patient voice. In the absence of options, women may think the pink ribbon approach is the only or the most appropriate to the disease. As a result, women may feel confused, limited, or ashamed of their feelings or actions concerning their breast cancer experiences if they don't choose the "pink" path. Ultimately, women's voices are potentially being silenced.

Pink ribbon rhetoric dominates the cultural construction of breast cancer. It is through the images and language of groups such as Komen that we learn to approach the disease in specific, pink-approved ways. As an example, one outcome of the pink ribbon movement's influence on behavior is the expectation that those diagnosed with breast cancer make specific choices, like publicly disclose their illnesses and maintain a positive attitude. This dismisses the voices of those who choose non-normative breast cancer experiences, like those who desire privacy or those who wish to bear witness to the painful realities of the disease.

Although the pink ribbon movement was born of a desire to remove stigma from breast cancer and provide voice, it has been established that some aspects of the movement perpetuate shame (Sulik, 2010). In this chapter I will build on this premise to argue that sponsors of women's breast healthcare who display support for the pink ribbon movement are implicated in the movement's shaming. Through a theoretical framework of shame (Kaufman, 1992; Lewis, 1987; Sontag, 1978), I outline the potential effects of specific pink ribbon artifacts on breast cancer patients' conceptions of self by problematizing the pink ribbon's presence in one location of women's breast healthcare: a patient waiting area connected to a mammography imaging room. I do this in an effort to extend popular critiques of the pink ribbon movement (King, 2008; Sulik, 2010). Finally, I will call for those connected to women's breast healthcare to more fully consider the implications of their support of the pink ribbon in relation to patient identity and shame, so that women can feel free to voice their own breast cancer experiences.

Shame As an Individual and Cultural Experience

I employ both Gershen Kaufman (1992) and Helen Block Lewis's (1987) theories of shame to examine the effects of the pink ribbon movement in one medical site. Major scholars of shame at a time when shame was ignored clinically, Kaufman and Lewis worked individually to make shame a more prominent topic of study in psychology and sociology by challenging, what Lewis calls, "a long-standing neglect of the subject" (p. xi). Kaufman explains that shame is a "multidimensional, multilayered experience," that every individual experiences to some degree (p. 191). He further argues that shame is also a cultural experience, where each group "has its own distinct sources as well as targets of shame" (p. 191). Clarifying the role of the self in shame, Lewis suggests that a central component of the shame experience is the "self in the eyes of the other," and argues that shame comes from the threat of disconnection, whether brought on by others or through our inner monologs (p. 15).

Interestingly, although both scholars connect shame to identity and conceptions of the self, Kaufman (1992) specifically employs a metaphor of illness in his description of the power of shame: "The inner experience of shame is like a sickness within the self, a sickness of the soul" (p. 6). He compares shame to a wound, suggesting that it may be made internally by the self, or it may come from an external entity, and the two are interconnected. Regardless of the source of the shame, however, the impact is the same and includes low self-esteem, insecurity, and self-doubt—all disturbing effects for women already facing significant physical trauma.

Both theorists conclude that shame is a complex and painful experience, initiated by feelings of inadequacy and threats to our connections with others, an experience that remains hidden within individuals and in our culture, generally. As shame is hidden in these spaces, so, too, is shame hidden in the pink ribbon movement. My goal is to uncover this hidden shame in relation to breast cancer patient identity and the promotion of the pink ribbon version of breast cancer in one specific location of women's breast healthcare.

Disciplining the Breast Cancer Experience

In the last three decades, breast cancer has attracted much public attention through an increase in advocacy groups (e.g., Susan G. Komen; Avon's Breast Cancer Crusade), nationally sponsored "awareness" (e.g., National Breast Cancer Awareness Month; National Metastatic Breast Cancer Awareness Day), and related pink products (e.g., the iconic pink ribbon as seen on anything from batteries to bags of flour to NFL uniforms). Given this level of exposure, the number of individuals who have donated to the movement, and the staggering number of breast cancer diagnoses each year—with over 230,000 new cases of invasive breast cancer in women in 2014 alone—nearly everyone has some connection to the pink ribbon ("How many women get breast cancer?" 2014).

What we now know as the pink ribbon movement began in the early 1990s as, simply, the breast cancer movement. The promotion of the traditional feminine image and the focus on normalizing the breast cancer experience fed the identity of the breast cancer movement and influenced its choice of symbol: the pink ribbon. Appointed the official badge of the breast cancer movement in the early 1990s, it reinforced the value placed on normalcy, which served to maintain the ethos of the movement (Sulik, 2011, pp. 45–46). However, what the attention to pinkness overshadows is the ways the normative behaviors and language authorized by the movement work to discipline those who don't enthusiastically take up the "good breast cancer patient" identity as dictated by the pink ribbon movement. Women who may not want to engage in the accepted narrative are pressured to conform by constant reminders (e.g., pink-sponsored objects in patient waiting rooms) that they are deviant when they don't maintain the correct pink ribbon identity—an ethos that shapes the cultural understanding of breast cancer. As Kaufman (1992) and Lewis (1987) would suggest, these women's sense of belonging to the dominant group is threatened. They may feel inadequate, as if they're experiencing breast cancer the wrong way by choosing a different route in their own illnesses. And even if these women don't want to be a part of the pink ribbon community, and don't want to take on any "pink" identity, they are still affected by the movement's powerful shaping of cultural expectations of the breast cancer experience.

Public shaming for non-normative breast cancer discourse is evident in many spaces. For example, Barbara Ehrenreich (2001) reports on her unsettling experience participating in an online breast cancer discussion board. To demonstrate her point that only "positive attitudes" and discourse that maintains the appropriate ethos are welcome in the pink ribbon community, she posted a comment entitled "angry" where she vented about her medical problems and, most boldly, critiqued the "sappy" pink ribbons representing the illness (pp. 43–53). Her comment was met with minimal support, but most of the responses criticized her negativity, with one commenter calling her bitter, and another insisting she immediately seek counseling to address her negative disposition. Here we see Kaufman's (1992) target of shaming: women who threaten the positive identity of the movement by critiquing the ultrafeminized pink ribbon or speaking freely about the difficult physical and emotional effects of breast cancer. Lewis (1987) would identify this tactic as "deliberate shaming" for the purposes of "severe punishment" (pp. 1–2).

Ehrenreich's (2001) experience, and the many similar experiences diagnosed women endure, demonstrate the group shaming of women who don't engage in the appropriate discourse of the pink ribbon community, leading to private shame. This unspoken need to discipline points to a fundamental flaw in the pink ribbon movement: What was established to erase stigma has a prominent role in keeping that shame alive. Though this irony has been pointed out by others, what has not been discussed in the literature is how women's healthcare perpetuates this shame. Given the often-intimate relationship between patients, practitioners, and locations of women's breast healthcare, it is necessary to interrogate the unspoken messages in these spaces. To reinforce my argument, I present a case study of pink-related artifacts in one setting of women's breast healthcare to suggest that texts promoting the pink ribbon have the potential to incite feelings of shame in patients as they navigate the formation of their breast cancer identities.

Narrative As a Tool for Instruction

As described above, one pink ribbon artifact identified in the patient suite was a copy of the popular *Chicken Soup* book series created for an audience of breast cancer patients entitled *Chicken Soup for the Breast Cancer Survivor's Soul: Stories to Support, Inspire, and Heal* (2006). This particular object may have been donated by a patient, provided free from the publisher, or gifted by one of the radiologists who reads the mammogram's resulting breast images. Surely the motivation of the giver was positive and the book was not meant as a tool of indoctrination, yet there are effects of the choice to display this particular book, especially for diagnosed women. More specifically, the stories included in this text serve to discipline its readers into a positive view of breast cancer. The introduction begins with the following message:

> Going through the experience of breast cancer is no picnic, but with loving support, helpful advice and the healing powers of laughter, it can be achieved. It is our fondest hope that you will be encouraged, buoyed, uplifted and instructed by the stories contained in this book. Other breast-cancer survivors wrote them for you—to bring you hope, to give you strength and courage. (p. xv)

The first paragraph clearly articulates that one goal of the text is for women to be *instructed* by the stories, and the teaching begins with an introduction to language common in dominant pink ribbon discourse, including terms such as "hope" and "strength." Further, under chapter titles such as "Gratitude" and "Courage," cancer is situated as a "gift," and the diagnosed are positioned as well-respected "survivors," evidence that this text models the expected message of the pink ribbon movement, fueling a culture of pride in survivorship and a positive view of breast cancer as something from which the diagnosed can benefit. These messages are communicated through individual stories that glorify the breast cancer experience and situate the diagnosed as one who overcomes the odds.

An effect of the value placed on sharing personal stories as demonstrated in *Chicken Soup for the Breast Cancer Survivor's Soul* (2006) is the increase in the number of diagnosed women taking their stories beyond circles of immediate friends and family to the public in the form of memoirs and blogs. In many of these scenarios (e.g., women publicly identifying as "survivors") the participants are pleased to be "role models" to others and enjoy being described with positive terms such as "fearless" and "inspiring"— labels typically assigned to women with breast cancer. However, the expectation that women take up this specific pink-ribbon role, which includes enthusiastic disclosure and maintenance of the pink ribbon code, places tremendous pressure on the diagnosed. It also reinforces the traditional gender role of caretaker. For example, if a woman subscribes to the pink ribbon narrative, she is disciplined to hide fear and pain when describing her experiences, or situate fear and pain strictly as opportunities for growth. Further, women are disciplined to find humor in the experience, or to make light of traumatic moments (e.g., the introduction's "picnic" metaphor). These choices relate to the role of caretaker because women may feel the need to strategically hide the emotional and physical discomfort of the disease for the benefit of loved ones. Standards such as these and others are modeled in the introduction above, and through the dozens of stories published in the *Chicken Soup* text, and may result in a hiding response by women who fear external shaming because of an "other" breast cancer performance (Lewis, 1987).

Another effect of the pink-inspired breast cancer narrative, as explained by Judy Segal (2007), is the proliferation of breast cancer myths. In her analysis of the genre of the breast cancer narrative, Segal finds that "personal breast cancer stories are one means of producing and maintaining ignorance about breast cancer" (p. 4). She further argues that the standard narrative reinforces normative behavior and that "[t]hese homogeneous stories [that follow a predicable narrative arc from diagnosis through treatment], suppress or replace other stories [through] which breast cancer might be queried and explored" (p. 4). When alternative breast cancer narratives are ignored, the pink ribbon lens is reinforced and those who want to share non-normative events are dismissed and their experiences, diminished, inciting internal shame.

Narratives such as those highlighted in the *Chicken Soup for the Breast Cancer Survivor's Soul* (2006) text serve to model pink ribbon-appropriate reactions to diagnosis, treatment, and life after breast cancer. Other versions of breast cancer narratives are certainly available through a variety of publication outlets, yet this is the framework represented in this location, which suggests to patients that the dominant pink ribbon discourse is the preferred approach for narrating one's experiences. It is troubling to think that women who may wish to take an approach similar to Ehrenreich's (2001), and express stories of frustration, grief, or hopelessness in this location, may be shamed by other patients, staff, or practitioners.

Problematizing "Survivor" and Illness Discourse

A second object in the mammography patient suite that reinforced the values of the pink ribbon movement was a document advertising the Avon "Walk for Breast Cancer." This midsized poster featured a series of smiling women in pink t-shirts walking under a banner that read "SURVIVOR." Beneath the image was information for donating to the cause or signing up for the event. The picture central to this poster fortified many values of the pink ribbon movement (e.g., maintaining one's feminine appearance, presenting a positive affect), but I will focus on the broader implications of the "survivor" discourse and expectation that diagnosed women take up that title.

Initially, the term *survivor* was strategically used to "de-stigmatize the disease and empower diagnosed women to take personal and collective action" (Sulik, 2010, pp. 34–35). Yet women who shun this metaphor and others like it are marked for not engaging in the sanctioned discourse of the pink ribbon. More disturbing is that women who do take on the title of "survivor" or "fighter" can experience stigma because of the associations of the terms themselves, connotations women often don't or won't consider (Garrison, 2007). Specifically, this particular problem with "survivor" and similar metaphors is that if a patient were to have the unfortunate recurrence, she might feel as though she wasn't a good enough "survivor" or "fighter." In "battling" the final stages of disease—which ultimately results in death—she would lose her title and potentially feel shame in her final months of life for not "working hard enough" to prevent the cancer's return.

Barbara Brenner, former director of Breast Cancer Action, explains another effect of the term: "For me, the term 'survivor' also carries a notion that I am not dead of breast cancer because I am somehow better or different from the hundreds of thousands of women who have died of the disease" (Brenner, 2003, n.p.). The rhetoric of "survivor" powerfully separates women with a history of breast cancer into categories of success: the haves and the have-nots (Kaiser, 2008). Lastly, and perhaps most dangerously, this language implies that breast cancer is something everyone can survive. This is simply not true. Currently, there are no proven ways to avoid recurrence, other than the general medical advice of living a healthy lifestyle (which can also be shame-inducing: see Yadlon, 1997).

As Susan Sontag argued in her 1978 book *Illness as Metaphor*, the language of a society has powerful effects and, in the case of disease, is responsible for a certain level of the guilt sick people experience. When we think of illnesses such as breast cancer as a punishment or curse (e.g., "she had such a bad life attitude—I'm not surprised she got sick") or a result of "poor" choices (e.g., "she terminated a pregnancy in her twenties—I hear that caused her cancer"), these metaphors and this language blame the patient for her illness. Therefore, a piece of the stigma attached to illness is a result of the language used to talk about it. Although the current pink ribbon discourse (e.g., "fighter," "survivor") may seem far from shaming in that it poses the patient as proactive in her treatment, the implications are troubling. As Garrison (2007) explains, women who choose not to use this language, whether they find it to be inappropriate or ineffective for their individual experience, are silenced. Such silencing is a continuation of the effects of the pink ribbon in spaces of women's breast healthcare.

The Pressure of Pink Ribbon "Community"

A final pink ribbon artifact present in the communal area was an album of pictures of office employees at a local Komen event. This object is perhaps the most threatening of the three texts I've isolated, in that it most strongly reinforces the pink ribbon framework as *the* accepted approach to breast cancer because of its personalization. Although the other documents—a copy of *Chicken Soup for the Breast Cancer Survivor's Soul* (2006) and posters advertising Avon's "Walk for Breast Cancer"—could be interpreted as general suggestions for how to engage breast cancer in this space, the images of desk staff, mammography technicians, radiologists, and office administrators participating in a pink ribbon event clearly send the message of a personal and local communal investment. Women with histories of breast cancer who see this book of photographs may think that, because the office takes part in this event, they should, too. Taken a step further, women may see these images and feel as though the message being sent is, "look at the steps we're making to participate on our day off; this is how committed we are to the cause, making it the most appropriate choice."

The collection of photos combines the overarching goals of the first two artifacts in that it serves to narrate one set of individuals' experiences interacting in the breast cancer community, like the *Chicken Soup* text, and it disciplines its audience to value the "survivor" discourse in that it presents images of men and women supporting those affected by breast cancer and who self-identify as "survivors." Yet it potentially has more power to influence than the first two because it is a personalized showing of "appropriate" behavior in this specific pink ribbon community instead of a broader, societal taking-up of the pink ribbon, as the other two demonstrate. Whereas the other texts included breast cancer narratives from strangers and images of strangers participating in a pink ribbon event, this sample of visual rhetoric includes familiar faces engaging in the values of the movement. And these faces don't just represent the office, but they represent the individuals who have cared for patients in their times of need, who have touched their bodies, and perhaps even been the deliverers of upsetting health updates. This extra layer of intimacy and connectedness intensifies the focus on the pink ribbon as demonstrated through the album.

Given the personal connection between this artifact and the patient, the risk for patient shame is likely increased. It is far more threatening to disagree with or critique the values of a familiar space as represented by an individual than to do the same of a general population as represented in the first two artifacts. Kaufman (1992) observes, in reference to hierarchical systems between individuals, that "it is the affect of contempt which partitions the inferior from the superior" (p. 241). Women who outwardly show that they don't see value in the office's participation in Komen events are at risk for contempt, which invites shaming. And as Lewis (1987) argues, one of the strongest shaming punishments a group can deliver is to make a member feel ostracized.

A Call to Action

The texts I've identified that represent the pink ribbon value system, ranging from a book to a poster to personalized pictures, individually and collectively increase the pressure on patients in this location of women's breast healthcare to participate in pink-appropriate activities and, more broadly, accept the pink ribbon approach to breast cancer for themselves. Kaufman (1992) argues that "scenes of shame are reenacted" in all groups (p. 202). Ironically, though locations of breast healthcare are meant to be comforting to and supportive of patients and allow for individual voicing of experiences, the presence of the pink ribbon is a threat to this and potentially "reenacts" scenes of shame for women who find the messages in these locations at odds with their breast cancer experiences. In the case of this specific location, patient agency is also a pertinent issue. Women with histories of breast cancer *must* get regular mammograms, sometimes every three to six months, and cannot avoid the patient suite where a pink ribbon framework persists, unless, that is, they are to find another provider. This is rarely an option for women with anything other than top-tier insurance coverage. Consequently, affected women are forced to seek breast healthcare in an environment that, for some, consistently renews feelings of shame for questioning or not choosing a pink ribbon framework to experience breast cancer. Their agency is removed and they are silenced.

I'd like to suggest that sponsors of women's healthcare, especially individuals employed in locations of breast healthcare, look closely at texts displayed in offices and artifacts generally made available for patient consumption. More specifically, I argue that professionals who work with patients with histories of breast cancer carefully interrogate the verbal or nonverbal message(s) they send in relation to "appropriate" responses to breast cancer. Although I believe that it is not the intention of breast healthcare providers to directly shame women under their care, they must still be aware of the potentially threatening rhetorical effects of the objects they exhibit in reception areas, patient suites, and treatment rooms. This includes what may be deemed "supportive" materials (e.g., pamphlets advertising wig clinics) that, nonetheless, are making statements about what should and shouldn't be considered valuable (e.g., maintaining one's feminine appearance) in a patient's experience with breast cancer.

As a parallel, I suggest that sponsors of breast healthcare take a more critical look at the pink ribbon movement, overall. I would encourage invested parties to peel away the layers of the pink, question the ethics of groups like Komen, and think purposefully about the meta-messages presented in the pink community. How does the suggestion that patients in this location participate in pink-sponsored events impact a patient's self-esteem, sense of self-worth, or voice? What problematic cultural constructions of femininity are administrative and medical staff reinforcing when they, for example, display pink-sponsored images of in-treatment, postmastectomy women wearing wigs and make-up while participating in a "race?" When the values of certain breast cancer patients don't align with the values of the space where they're seeking medical assistance, and patients don't have the option of medical intervention from alternative sites, how does this impact the patient? In what ways can the site of care address the identity needs of all patients, including those who don't subscribe to the values of the pink ribbon movement? Questions like these can guide breast healthcare sponsors toward a responsible understanding of the pink ribbon movement, its effects, and the breast cancer identities and voices of the women they treat in their offices. As Kaufman (1992) notes, individuals need to feel "valued and respected," and when these needs are not provided for, "shame will inevitably ensue" (p. 201). Shame has no place in locations of breast healthcare.

References

Brenner, B. (2003, January 2). Please don't call me a survivor. *Chicago Tribune*. Retrieved from http://articles.chicagotribune.com/2003-01 02/news/0301020211_1_breast-cancer-cure-survivor.

Canfield, J., Hansen, M. V., Kelly, M. O. (2006). *Chicken soup for the breast cancer survivor's soul*. Deerfield Beach, FL: Health Communications.

Ehrenreich, B. (2001, November). Welcome to cancerland: A mammogram leads to a cult of pink kitsch. *Harper's Magazine*, 43–53.

Garrison, K. (2007). The personal is rhetorical: War, protest, and peace in breast cancer narratives. *Disability Studies Quarterly, 27*(4), 1–13.

"How many women get breast cancer?" (2014 September). *cancer.org*. Learn about cancer. Retrieved from http://www.cancer.org/cancer/breastcancer/overviewguide/breast-cancer-overview-key-statistics.

Kaiser, K. (2008). The meaning of survivor identity for women with breast cancer. *Social Science and Medicine, 67*(1), 79–87.

Kaufman, G. (1992). *The power of caring*. Rochester, VT: Schenkman Books.

King, S. (2006). Pink ribbons inc.: Breast cancer and the politics of philanthropy. Minneapolis: University of Minnesota Press.

Lewis, H. B. (1987). *The role of shame in symptom formation*. Hillsdale, NJ: Lawrence Erlbaum.

Segal, J. (2007). Breast cancer narratives as public rhetoric: Genre itself and the maintenance of ignorance. *Linguistics and the Human Sciences, 3*(1), 3–23.

Sontag, S. (1978). *Illness as metaphor*. New York: Farrar, Straus & Giroux.

Sulik, G. (2010). Pink ribbon blues: How breast cancer culture undermines women's health. Oxford: Oxford University Press.

Yandlon, S. (1997). Skinny women and good mothers: The rhetoric of risk, control, and culpability in the production of knowledge about breast cancer. *Feminist Studies, 23*(3), 645–677.

Section III

Make It Taboo

Motherhood, Mothering, and Reproduction

5 Giving Voice to Women's Childbirth Preferences

Edith LeFebvre and Carmen Stitt

One of the most life-changing events a woman can experience is becoming pregnant and giving birth. Giving birth is a natural phenomenon, often stressful during the 39–42 weeks of gestation because of the many changes, both emotionally and physically, that a pregnant woman must grapple with while moving toward the process of delivery. This chapter identifies and examines current birthing practices offered by many hospitals primarily but not exclusively, found in the United States.

Background and History

Over the past one hundred years, the practice of women giving birth in the United States has shifted from becoming a natural occurrence in the home, predominantly attended by laypersons or midwives, to being treated as an increasingly medical phenomenon. By the mid-20th century, options for delivery had developed to offer hospital care resulting in more live births and with maternal mortality rates decreasing (Zwelling, 2008). The sterile accommodations and twilight sleep were welcomed as modern and desirable. At the same time, women's dependence on the medical community to supervise their pregnancy and labor was established as the norm.

Gradually, the inclusion of advanced miracle pharmaceuticals to ease the pain of childbirth and induce labor, and the use of technology, were perceived by most as the only reasonable option to ensure a healthy delivery. What initially may have appeared as contemporary and safe birthing practices resulted in altering the process of giving birth, turning it into a complicated, risky, and unnatural experience. In fact, as medical technology has advanced, so has the increase in intervention-intensive labor and birth, along with women's fear of labor or belief in their ability to cope with the pain of childbirth (Romano & Lothian, 2007). Zwelling (2008) found that some obstetricians actually frightened their nulliparous patients and that one woman obstetrician reportedly explained to her pregnant patient that "labor is barbaric" (p. 89).

Medically managed labor and delivery require most women to remain in bed in a supine position, which prohibits natural movement during labor as they are connected to an intravenous line and fetal monitor. Giving birth in a supine position does not facilitate giving birth naturally and most often prolongs labor (Gupta, Hofmeyr, & Smyth, 2004). Restricting movement while providing drugs that contradict a body's natural labor process is often counterproductive and may contribute to unplanned Cesarean surgery.

The reasons for a shift from a naturalistic human experience to more of a medical model are many. Although birthing is a "natural" function of the body, it is not without risks to the mother and child. Some contemporary preferences for childbirth favor a predictable and neat outcome to "fit" with modern lifestyles (Mazzoni et al., 2010). In many cases, this includes surgical procedures for birth even though they are not medically necessary, such as routine episiotomies and Cesareans. Technology that can save a woman and her newborn's lives has also greatly improved, providing life-saving capabilities, which have not otherwise been available. However, the previous century saw a rise in medically assisted births not witnessed before, and not necessarily medically indicated. It is for this reason we examine how and why historical practices have changed, and how these changes impact communication between women and medical professionals about birthing options.

Beginning in the late 1800s, as anesthesia and antiseptics were increasingly accepted, so too was Cesarean surgery (CS), whereby fetuses are delivered with the assistance of a surgeon slicing through the mother's abdomen. CS has become more commonly used since the 1970s (Natcher, 2011). In 1970, 5% of all births were done by CS. As CS rates began to rise, the World Health Organization (WHO) stated, "There is no justification for any region to have CS rates higher than 10–15%" (World Health Organization, 2008b). By 2009, the CS rate skyrocketed to 32.9% (VBAC, 2013), and now CS rates have stabilized at 32% (Center for Disease Control and Prevention, 2014; Declercq, 2010; Hendrickson, 2012). Although a boon to medically necessary cases where the mother's or the fetus's life is at risk, the procedure of CS carries its own risk that may not be completely explained or revealed prior to elective CS deliveries.

Risks of CS to the mother include infection, blood loss, blood clots in the legs, pelvic organs, and lungs, injury to the bowel and bladder, and possible reactions to the anesthesia used (http://www.acog.org/Patients/FAQs/Cesarean-Birth#complications). Longer term risks to the mother include breaking open of the incision during subsequent labor and delivery, placenta previa, placenta accreta, placenta increta, and placenta percreta. These risks to the mother increase with each subsequent CS delivery. Risks to the infant include injury during delivery, need for care after delivery in a neonatal intensive care unit, and breathing problems (American Congress of Obstetricians and Gynecologists, 2011). Paradoxically, the increase in CS rates is not associated with a corresponding decrease in morbidity and mortality for mother and child (McCourt et al., 2007). The risk for postpartum maternal death is 3.6 times higher for women who have

CS compared to those who deliver vaginally (Denuex-Tharaux, Carmona, Bouvier-Colle, & Breart, 2006).

Minority women are in a unique position when it comes to CS. Some minority women in the US are more likely to have CS compared to Caucasians. Among minorities in the United States, African Americans, Puerto Ricans, and American Indian/Alaskan Natives are more likely than whites to have CS (Getahun et al., 2009; Declercq, 2010; Braveman, Egerter, Edmonston, & Verdon, 1995). Some have speculated that differences in CS rates may be attributed to insurance types; however, several studies have shown that after adjusting for other risk factors, private and publicly insured women were equally likely to undergo CS (Haque, Faysel, & Khan, 2010; Movsas, Wells, Mongoven, & Grigorescu, 2012). Nonetheless, a comparative study of uninsured Nevada women found them less likely to undergo CS than women with insurance (Shen & Wei, 2012). The increase in CS presents a vexing social problem. On the one hand, minority women, like their Caucasian counterparts, are able to elect a delivery method to fit their preferences as much as their white counterparts. On the other hand, having higher CS rates, even as elective surgery, presents its own risks to women and newborns, as discussed earlier. Given that patient education is critical to making informed decisions during a pregnancy and the delivery, coupled with potential or indirect influences by medical personnel who support CS, women need to be educated about the risks from CS.

Of the women who choose to have CS, often many psychological, sociological, and cultural reasons explain how they came to elect CS. Several studies have shown that women obtain information about the birthing process from a variety of sources, including friends and family members, medical professionals, and the media (Miller & Shriver, 2012). Frequently, women don't use this information in order to make an informed choice, but rather, to confirm previously held beliefs. Women selectively consult outsides sources that confirm their beliefs and then refute those sources that don't. Consequently, informed consent no longer exists because the process of objectively weighing costs and benefits of procedures does not occur. These findings have been corroborated in several studies of patients who were not in favor of CS, but were anxious about the process of birth. After consulting their medical professionals, women were persuaded by their physicians to select CS to alleviate their anxiety over pain during delivery (Goldberg & Shorten, 2014; Hopkins, 2000; Malacrida & Boulton, 2014).

Most recent data show that the United States ranks 29th in the world on infant mortality, tied with Poland and Slovakia (National Center for Health Statistics, 2007). More disturbingly, CS rates were 2.4 times higher for African American women than for Caucasian women, with rates of Puerto Rican and American Indian/Alaskan Natives infant mortality rates similarly elevated above Caucasians (MacDorman & Mathews, 2008). We will now look at other aspects of the modern birthing process to explain why CS rates have continued to increase.

In current practices, hospitals treat delivery as a medical procedure. Coupling that approach with a business perspective, hospitals are decidedly risk averse. At the first sign of trouble, the line of defense taken is to prepare for the worst. Frequently, that includes CS. As obstetrician Jeffrey Ecker noted in an interview, hospitals and doctors don't typically get sued for CS. "They do get sued for not intervening" (Lake, 2012, para. 17). Yet it is not risk aversion or medical practice alone that drives the increase in CS rates.

In a very complicated insurance and reimbursement procedure in the United States, medical professionals are reimbursed by procedure rather than on an hourly basis. Medical professionals get paid the same whether they deliver a baby in 48 or 12 hours. One analysis of California hospitals found that women who deliver in for-profit hospitals were 15% more likely to deliver by CS than women who gave birth in nonprofit hospitals (Johnson, 2010). Moreover, a hospital stands to make as much as twice the profit from a CS compared to a vaginal delivery. Some sources estimate the cost of a vaginal delivery at $10,100 compared to $23,111 for a CS delivery—a $10,000 difference (U.S. Department of Health and Human Services, 2010). The cost range, however, depends on geographic location. On average in the US, CS delivery costs $8856 compared to a vaginal delivery $6152, a $2704 difference (CAREOperatives, 2013). It would be a stretch to suggest hospitals openly direct a woman's birth plans for delivery. Nonetheless, it is suggested that there are more subtle ways for medical facilities to influence medical professionals, who in turn influence their patients to consider CS, such as recommending a higher turnover in beds (Johnson, 2010).

Hospitals and insurance reimbursement rates aren't the only factors contributing to the rise in CS. The improvements in technology and the ease with which medical procedures can be carried out also make CS an outwardly appealing choice for a minority of women. Studies show that of the CS performed some women request to have CS that are elective (not medically necessary). However, among the medical community, the debate surrounding the rates and appropriateness of maternal requests for CS versus CS carried out for other reasons is ongoing.

In response to a 2006 state-of-the-science conference convened by the National Institutes of Health, one doctor noted in reaction to the rising CS rates "that it was mothers themselves who asked for the surgical procedure is unadulterated fraud" (Peralta personal comment as quoted in Young, 2006, p. 6). Countering that claim, a national poll of mothers in the United States who had a CS during 2011–2012 found that maternal-requested Cesarean surgeries were *"infrequent,"* with only 1% reporting they requested a CS for nonmedical reasons (Childbirth Connection, 2013). Thus, maternal requests for CS do occur but are only a minor factor explaining the high CS rates. The medical organization practicing empiricallybased medicine is certainly aware of the high rates of CS among women in the United States and very recently took steps to reduce it, yet its official position on CS is equivocal at best.

A short time ago, the leading professional organizations of medical doctors treating women, the American College of Obstetricians and Gynecologists (ACOG) and the Society for Maternal-Fetal Medicine (SMFM), jointly issued a statement to reduce the CS rate among first-time mothers (American Congress of Obstetricians and Gynecologist, 2014). The onus was on the doctors to balance the risk–benefit ratio for an otherwise healthy mother and child when deciding whether to perform a CS. However, guiding doctors is ACOG's official (and contradictory) committee position dated April 2013. In its report, ACOG highlights the "potential short-term benefits of planned cesarean compared with planned vaginal delivery (including women who give birth vaginally and those who choose cesarean in labor)." (American Congress of Obstetricians and Gynecologist, 2013). CS was *not* recommended prior to 39 weeks gestation, "in the absence of effective pain management" or "for women desiring several children" (ACOG Committee Opinion #559, p. 1). Professional organizations have left the door open for performing a medical procedure that is not medically necessary, which may limit women's voices in the delivery room and may contribute to the high CS rate.

Other practices among modern medical birthing procedures help to create an atmosphere limiting women's voices in order for medical facilities to keep an "efficient business" rather than allow women to birth more naturally (Lake, 2012).

Many hospitals encourage and/or insist on administering pharmaceuticals that cease or delay contractions and cervix dilation during labor. Women who give birth in hospitals are routinely hooked up to continuous electronic fetal monitoring (EFM) and given epidurals in case a CS is needed (Lake, 2012). Medical care givers often manipulate women through their language choices during labor, leading them to believe their infant is experiencing "fetal distress," so that anything other than a natural birth experience becomes mandatory.

The legal climate is such that hospitals encourage their medical staff to prepare for CS. Although common sense dictates this would be a "best practice," one needs to bear in mind that setting up women for a medical procedure that they likely will not need exposes the mother and infant to unnecessary risks. The World Health Organization estimates that in 2008, 6.20 million unnecessary Cesarean surgeries were performed (World Health Organization, 2008). Racial disparities were found to exist between those who have CS and those who do not.

A recent retrospective study of over 11,000 hospital births replicated previous findings showing that African Americans are more likely to undergo CS than their White counterparts due to nonreassuring fetal heart tracings (Washington, Caughey, Cheng, & Bryant, 2011). However, unlike other studies, the researchers had access to other patient data that might confound results, such as body mass index and obstetrical and medical information. They concluded that based on these findings, a nonreassuring fetal heart rate is a relatively subjective measure with lower interrater reliability (Chauhan, Klauser, Woodring, et al. 2008) and that practitioner bias relating to minorities' risk factors and legal implications could enter into the equation when deciding to perform a CS. Unfortunately, at this point in the labor process, after hours of intrusive care that fails to enhance delivery, CS is often indicated as the only viable way of giving birth.

Although today both medical professionals and patients can easily find information regarding the short- and long-term potential of negative effects of CS, women and their doctors continue to elect birthing practices that are not ideal for their newborns. The CS rate continues apace and seemingly without realization of the domino effect CS deliveries have on a newborn or on a woman's body. A small portion of women voluntarily decide to have CS for a variety of reasons, including fear of pain during the delivery process (Bourgeault et al., 2008), concerns about the effects of pushing on one's pelvic floor during delivery, consequent potential incontinence, and the sheer convenience of being able to predict and time delivery (Wax, Cartin, Pinette, & Blackstone, 2004). Many women believe that after having a CS subsequent deliveries must also be by CS, but this is not the case. On the contrary, a National Institutes of Health (2004) study concluded that risks to women and their newborns with vaginal birth after Cesarean (VBAC) are low. However, most women are not receiving this information.

Recent studies show that women are not being informed either about the risks of CS or the benefits of having a VBAC (Bernstein, Matalon-Grazi, & Rosenn, 2012). Exacerbating the problem are patients' perception that a doctor prefers a CS, in which case patients do not assert themselves to inquire about trying a vaginal birth after CS (Bernstein et al., 2012). The combination of these conditions sets the stage, in effect, for silencing the patient when birth choices are made.

Pharmaceuticals in the Delivery Room and Effects

Unfortunately, as hospitals became the predominant choice for labor and delivery, a medical-surgical model of care became rooted. In hospital settings, doctors frequently administer synthetic hormones or otherwise artificially interfere with delivery in order to stimulate contractions. This common practice in hospitals is found to be associated with higher CS rates (Lake, 2010). The model of care that relies upon pharmaceuticals leads to separation of mother and newborn at birth to prevent infection; as a result of this separation, there is a decrease in breastfeeding: With birth considered a pathological event, the mother requires rest and hospitalization (Pitcock & Clark, 1992). Moreover, following a CS delivery a new mother often is taking pain medication that may prevent her from breastfeeding because of the potential crossover of the drug into her milk. Women who do not breastfeed miss out on the numerous benefits not only to the child, but to themselves as well.

Breastfeeding lowers a woman's risk of heart attack and stroke (Schwartz et al., 2010), decreases her risk of breast and ovarian cancer, and makes it more likely for her to resume her prepregnancy weight more quickly than women who do not breastfeed (LaLeche League, 2007). Benefits to newborns include increased immunity to disease, less mortality due to sudden infant death dyndrome (SIDS), as well as long-term effects such as increased IQ, less likelihood of obesity, half the likelihood of ear infections during the first year of life, less chance of allergies, asthma, eczema, and many other benefits. With all of these benefits, one wonders why information linking vaginal delivery with breastfeeding and positive outcomes for mother and child is not given out when the topic of CS comes up.

When women are not made aware of the differences in the benefits of giving natural childbirth in comparison to CS, and/or CS is promoted or directed by managed care providers, making an informed decision becomes impossible. Thus, following a CS, bonding between mother and infant is postponed, resulting in the infant not receiving the numerous benefits that only mother's milk provides newborns (Pitcock & Clark, 1992).

Rising to the prominence of policy and practice in hospitals, contemporary delivery approaches often prove to negatively affect the natural process of giving birth. Some medical personnel were not exposed during training to normal birthing practices and/or the problems associated with use of contemporary interventions. Many medical personnel have been taught that the status quo is policy aimed at easing the delivery for the mother, safe guarding the infant, and protecting the doctor and hospital from malpractice suits. However, many nulliparous women considered low-risk are seldom educated about alternative birth or natural delivery choices at a level that would allow them to make an informed choice. Many of these women are then caught in the web of terror during the birth process and in many contemporary hospital deliveries. These women accept a barrage of treatment and monitoring that often leave them feeling depressed and physically abused (Goer, Leslie, & Romano, 2007). The unnatural and intrusive care some of these women receive takes place in hospitals whose policies have been constructed to place economics, personnel convenience, and liability management ahead of best practices for mother and infant.

One protocol that is often used for convenience or for nonmedical indications by medical caretakers or requested by patients is the induction of labor. Rather than spontaneous labor, elective induction is generally a precursor for analgesia, epidural anesthesia, and neonatal resuscitation and Cesarean surgeries, and may increase the likelihood of instrumental vaginal delivery, intrapartum fever, shoulder dystocia, low birth weight, and admission of the newborn to the neonatal intensive care unit (Goer et al., 2007; Romano & Lathian, 2007).

Given the serious medical consequences of an elective induction, it is difficult to comprehend why induction without medical indications is promoted or allowed, except that it does support current hospital practice and policy. Declercq, Sakala, Corry, and Applebaum (2006) found that labor was induced in 34% of all live births in 2005. A lack of information and/ or education provided to women, coupled with a sense of trust in hospital care, medical professionals, and perceived safety offered by advanced technology and available pharmaceuticals, have left many women with regrets and physical harm following their medically managed birthing experience (Malacrida & Boulton, 2014).

Conclusion

Many women in the United States in the 21st century have taken full advantage of the purported medical and technological advances made available to them in relation to birthing practices. We live in an era when seemingly unlimited information is available at one's fingertips. However, many women buy into the predominant belief that birthing a newborn is something to fear, that it cannot be completed unless it is medically attended, and that one's own body cannot do it without medical intervention. For the majority of women who will give birth without complications, these medical and technological advances are not necessarily better for either their own or their newborn's health. What can women do to change this trajectory?

We suggest that a starting point lies with the very people who are at the heart of the issue: women. When women tell their birth stories, these are experiences filled with a range of emotions and keen insight from first-hand experience. These insights are rich in information that we believe needs to drive the conversation of modern-day birthing practices, given an absence of medical complication during a pregnancy. The birth process for the new mother can be frightening: The very loss of control of one's body as labor begins may leave a woman vulnerable as she relies on the experience and knowledge of the healthcare professionals ministering to her. Unfortunately, that trust may be misplaced.

The past century saw an unprecedented rise in medical knowledge and technology. No woman would likely forego medical intervention in the event that either her own or her fetus's life was at risk or in danger. This chapter, however, addresses the majority of births that occur without complications; the overwhelming majority of complications are known well in advance of the onset of labor. Pregnant women, in particular, can be distinguished from other "patients" in their need for the latest medical interventions because their lives, and the lives of their newborn, are at stake. As indicated in this chapter, when it comes to medical intervention with low-risk pregnancies, more is not always better. In some cases, it is worse. As tantalizing as it is to take advantage of the latest medicine and technology, and most assuredly, to experience the least amount of pain, many women have followed the pied piper of medical advances. In doing so, they have left behind the more human-centered approaches to childbirth and often their voice in the decision-making process as well.

What was once commonplace, midwifery, has been pushed off to the fringes of society. Despite insurance coverage, fewer than 9% of all births in the United States are attended by midwives (midwife.org). According to the American College of Nurse-Midwives, trained and certified midwives are covered by Medicaid in all 50 states, and the majority of states mandate private insurance reimbursement for midwifery services (midwife.org) In many ways, midwives are in competition with the obstetrics practice. One wonders why there are not more conversations about the disparities in health outcomes for minorities and the options available for less invasive, more women-direct birthing experiences.

Women's birth experiences can be powerful from a variety of perspectives and in subtle ways. Often, women are overwhelmed with the very real circumstances they find themselves in after giving birth, and the inordinate amount of time required to care for a newborn and to recover both physically and emotionally. After all, what matters to a new mother is that the baby is healthy and cared for. Women lose sight of what seemed like small frustrations in the hospital that occurred during labor or delivery, but that they *wished* had gone differently. These frustrations may stem from communication strategies between women and medical professionals manifested during labor and delivery, but a mother frequently discounts the importance of these frustrations following birth. It is these frustrations generated from the differences between women's voiced preferences and the policies of medical professionals or managed care that we have sought to underscore here. *These* are the very voices that get lost after a newborn comes along.

Similarly, women who opt to give birth in "nontraditional" ways—such as using a midwife in a hospital setting, using a doula (a person hired to attend and carry out a mother's birth plan so that the mother can focus on herself and the birth of her fetus), or using freestanding birthing clinics attended by trained and certified midwives—can lend a strong voice promoting a more humanistic approach to birthing practices. These women's experiences can be life-changing and when voiced can help other women decide on the best birth options for them. It is a woman's right to choose how to give birth.

By raising their voices and obtaining complete information on all the birth options and birth experiences available, in addition to a hospital's managed care approach, women need not feel compelled to ignore their preferences. Rather, as more women's voices address the reality of the current managed care practice of birth, women can be empowered to make more informed choices about what is right for themselves.

References

American Congress of Obstetricians and Gynecologists. (2011, May). Cesarean birth. *Frequently Asked Questions: Labor, Delivery and Postpartum Care.* Retrieved from http://www.acog.org/Patients/FAWs/Cesarean-Birth#complications.

American Congress of Obstetricians and Gynecologists. (2013, April). Cesarean delivery on maternal request. *Committee Opinion No. 559*, 1. Retrieved from http://www.acog.org/Resources_And_Publications/Committee_Opinions/Committee_on_Obstetric_Practice/Cesarean_Delivery_on_Maternal_Request.

American Congress of Obstetricians and Gynecologists. (2014, February 19). Nation's ob-gyns take aim at preventing cesareans. Retrieved from http://www.acog.org/About-ACOG/News-Room/News-Releases/2014/Nations-Ob-Gyns-Take-Aim-at-Preventing-Cesareans.

Bernstein, S. N., Matalon-Grazi, P. A., & Rosenn, M. (2012). Trial of labor versus repeat cesarean: Are patients making an informed decision? *American Journal of Obstetrics and Gynecology*, 204–207, e1–6.

Bourgeault, I. L., Declercq, E., Sandall, J., Wrede, S., Vanstone, M., van Teijlingen, E., Devries, R., & Benoit, C. (2008). Too posh to push? Comparative perspectives on maternal request Cesarean sections in Canada, the U.S., the U.K., and Finland. *Advances in Medical Sociology*, 10, 99–123.

Braveman, P., Egerter, S., Edmonston, F., & Verdon, M. (1995). Racial/ethnic differences in the likelihood of Cesarean delivery, California. *American Journal of Public Health*, 85, 625–630.

CAREOperatives. (2013). *Healthcare Blue Book: Cesarean section delivery*. Retrieved online January 23, 2013, from: http://healthcarebluebook.com/pageResults.aspx?id=107&dataset=MD.

Center for Disease Control and Prevention. (2014, February 25). Births: Methods of delivery. Hyattsville, MD: National Center for Health Statistics. Retrieved from http:www.cdc.gov/nchs/fastats/delivery.htm.

Chauhan, S. P., Klauser, C. K., Woodring, T. C., et al. (2008). Intrapartum nonreassuring fetal heart rate tracing and prediction of adverse outcomes: Interobserver variability. *American Journal of Obstetrics Gynecology*, 199, 623 e1–5.

Childbirth Connection. (2012). *Why is the national U.S. Cesarean section rate so high?* New York: Childbirth Connection.

Childhood Connection. (2013). *National Institutes of Health: Interpreting meeting and media reports. Alerts and Responses*. New York: Childbirth Connection.

Coleman-Cowger, E. H., Erikson, K., Spong, C. Y., Portnoy, B., Croswell, J., & Schulkin, J. (2010). Current practice of Cesarean delivery on maternal request following the 2006 state-of-the-science conference. *Journal of Reproductive Medicine*, 55(1–2), 25–30.

Declercq, E. R. (2010, February 3). *The causes and consequence of disparities by race/ethnicity in Cesarean section rates*. Boston: Boston University School of Public Health.

Declercq, E. R., Sakala, C., Corry, M. P., & Applebaum, S. (2006). *Listening to mothers II: Report of the second national U.S. survey of women's childbearing experiences*. New York: Childbirth Connection.

Deneux-Tharaux, C., Carmona, E., Bouvier-Colle, H., & Breart, G. (2006, September). Postpartum maternal mortality and Cesarean delivery. *Obstetrics and Gynecology*, 108 (3 Pt 1), 541–548. Retrieved from http:www.ncbi.nlm.nih.gov/pubmed/16946213.

Ericssen, L. M., Ellen, A. N., & Hanne Kjaergaard, R. M. (2011, December). Mode of delivery after epidural analgesia in a cohort of low-risk nulliparas. *Birth: Issues in perinatal care*, 38(4), 317–326.

Fuglenes, D., Aas, E., Botten, G., Oian, P., & Kristiansen, I. S. (2012). Maternal preference for Cesarean delivery: Do women get what they want? *American College of Obstetricians and Gynecologists*, 120(2), 252–260.

Gallagher, F., Bell, L., Waddell, G., Benoit, A., & Cote, N. (2012, March). Requesting Cesareans without medical indications: An option being considered by young Canadian women. *Birth, 39*, 39–47.

Getahun, D., Strickland, D., Lawrence, J. M., Fassett, M. J., Koebnick, C., & Jacobsen, S. J. (2009, October). Racial and ethnic disparities in the trends in primary cesarean delivery based on indications. *American Journal of Obstetrics and Gynecology, 201*, 422.e1–422.e7.

Goer, H., Leslie, M. S., & Romano, A. (2007). The coalition for improving maternity services: Evidence basis for the ten steps of mother-friendly care: Step 6: Does not routinely employ practice, procedures unsupported by scientific evidence. *Journal of Perinatal Education, 16*(1), 32S–64S.

Goldberg, H. B., & Shorten, A. (2014). Patient and provider perceptions of decision making about use of epidural analgesia during childbirth: A thematic analysis. *Journal of Perinatal Education, 23*(3), 142–150.

Gupta, J. K., Hofmeyr, G. J., & Smyth R. (2004). Position in the second stage of labour for women without epidural anaesthesia. *Cochrane Database of Systematic Reviews* (1). DOI: 10.1002/14651858.CD002006.pub2.

Hamilton, B. E., Martin, J. A., & Ventura, S. J. (2012, October 3). Births: Preliminary data for 2011. *National Vital Statistics Reports, 61*(5).

Haque, S. S., Faysel, M. A., & Khan, H. M. R. (2010). Racial differences in the use of most commonly performed medical procedures in the United States. *Journal of Health Disparities Research and Practice, 4*(1), 14–25.

Hendrickson, K. (2012, March 28). *Cesarean sections in the U.S.: The trouble with assembling evidence from data.* Retrieved online January 23, 2013, from: http://blogs.scientificamerican.com/guest-blog/2012/03/28/cesarean-sections-in-the-u-s-the-trouble-with-assembling-evidence-from-data.

Hodges, S. (2006, March). The politics of women's health; Maternal request for Cesarean delivery: Myth or reality. *Our bodies ourselves.* Boston: Boston Women's Health Book Collective.

Hopkins K. (2000). Are Brazilian women really choosing to deliver by Cesarean? *Social Science Medicine, 5*(1), 725–740.

Horey, D., Weaver, J., & Russell, H. (2004). Information for pregnant women about Cesarean birth. *Cochrane Database System Review* (1): CD003858.

Johnson, N. (2010, September 9). *Cesarean sections: Increasing and profitable.* Retrieved online January 23, from http://kalwnews.org/audio/2010/09/02/cesarean-sections-increasing-and-profitable 565229.html.

Lake, N. (2012). Labor Interrupted. *Harvard Magazine.* Retrieved February 2, 2013, from: http://harvardmagazine.com/2012/11/labor-interrupted.

La Leche League International. (2007, October 14). *What are the benefits of breast-feeding my baby?* Retrieved February 12, 2013, from http://www.lalecheleague.org/nb/nbbenefits.html.

Lieberman, E. & O'Donoghue, C. (2002). Unintended effects of epidural analgesia during labor: A systematic review. *American Journal of Obstetrics and Gynecology, 186*, S31–S68.

Martin, J. A., Hamilton, B. E., Sutton, P. D., Ventura, S. J., Matthews, T. J., Kirmeyer, S. (2010). Births: Final data for 2007. *National Vital Statistics Reports, 58*(24), 1–85.

MacDorman, M. R., & Mathews, M. S. (2008). Recent trends in infant mortality in the United States. *NCHS Data Brief, 9.* Retrieved October 15, 2015, from http://www.cdc.gov/nchs/data/databriefs/db09.htm.

MacKenzie, Bryers, H,. & van Teijlingen, E (2010, October). Risk, theory, social and medical models: A critical analysis of the concept of risk in maternity care. *Midwifery, 26*(5): 488–496.

Malacrida, C., & Boulton, T., (2014). The best laid plans? Women's choices, expectations and experiences in childbirth. *Health 18*(1), 41–59.

Mazzoni, A., Althabe, F., Liu, N. H., Bonotti, A. M., Gibbons, L., Sanchez, A. J. & Belizan, J. M. (2010, December 7). Women's preference for Caesarean section: A systematic review and meta-analysis of observational studies. *BJOG, 118*, 391–399. DOI: 10.1111/j.1471-0528.2010.02793.x. Retrieved October 12, 2015, from http://onlinelibrary.wiley.com.proxy.lib.csus.edu.

McCourt, C., Weaver, J., Statham, H., Beakes, S., Gamble, J., & Creedy, D. K. (2007). Elective Cesarean section and decision making: A critical review of the literature. *Birth, 34*(1), 65–79.

Miller, A. C., & Shriver, T. E. (2012). Women's childbirth preferences and practices in the United States. *Social Science Medicine, 75*(4): 709–716.

Movsas, T., Z., Wells, E., Mongoven, A., & Grigorescu, V. (2012). Does medical insurance type (private vs public) influence the physician's decision to perform Caesarean delivery? *Journal of Medical Ethics, 38*, 470–473.

Munroe, S. , Kornelsen, J., & Hutton, E. (2009, September–October). Decision making in patient-initiated elective Cesarean delivery: The influence of birth stories. *Social Science Medicine, 34*(5): 373–379.

Murphy, K., Grabman, W. A., Todd, A. L., & Holl, J. L. (2007, December). Association between rising professional liability insurance premiums and primary Cesarean delivery rates. *American College of Obstetricians and Gynecologists, 110*(6), 1264–1268.

Natcher, W. H. (2011, April 8). *NIH state-of-the-science conference: Cesarean U.S.* National Library of Medicine. National Institute of Health. Retrieved January 23, 2013, from: www.nih.gov.

National Center for Health Statistics. (2007). *Health, United States, 2007 with chartbook on trends in the health of Americans*. Hyattsville, MD: National Center for Health Statustics.

National Institute of Health. (2004, December 14). *Risks from labor after prior Cesarean delivery low, study reports*. Retrieved February 10, 2013, from: http://www.nih.gov/news/pr/de2004/nichd-14.htm.

Pitcock, P. C., & Clark, R. B. (1992). From Fanny to Fernard: The development of consumerism in pain control during the birth process. *American Journal of Obstetrics and Gynecology, 167*, 581–587.

Prior, E., Santhakumaran, S., Gale, C., Philipps, L. H., Modi, N., & Hyde, M. J. (2012, April 23). Breastfeeding after Cesarean delivery: A systematic review and meta-analysis of world literature. *American Journal of Clinical Nutrition.* Retrieved February 2, 2013, from: www.AJCN.org.

Romano, A. M., & Lothian, J. A. (2007). Promoting, protecting, and supporting normal birth: A look at the evidence. *Journal of Obstetrics, Gynecology and Neonatal Nursing, 37*, 94–105. DOI: 10.111/J. 15526809.2007.00210.

Schwartz, E. B., McClure, C. K., Tepper, P. G., Thurston, R., Janssen, I., Matthews, K. A., & Sutton-Tyrrell, K. (2010). Lactation and maternal measures of subclinical cardiovascular disease. *American College of Obstetricians and Gynecologists, 115*(1): 41–48.

Shen, J. J., & Wei, H. (2012). Adverse maternal outcomes for women with different health insurance statuses in Nevada. *Nevada Journal of Public Health, 5*(1), 38–45.

Smith, L. J. (2010, December 24). Impact on birthing practices on the breastfeeding dyad. *Journal of Midwifery and Women's Health,52*(6), 621–630.

Stafford, R. S. (1990, March). Cesarean section use and source of payment: An analysis of California hospital discharge abstracts. *American Journal of Public Health, 80*(3), 313–315.

Stevens, G., & Miller, Y. D. (2012, September 3). Overdue choices: How information and role in decision-making influence women's preferences for induction for prolonged pregnancy. *Birth, 39*, 248–257.

U.S. Census Bureau (2012). Births, deaths, marriages, and divorces. *Statistical abstract of the United States.* Washington, DC: United States Census Bureau.

U.S. Department of Health and Human Services. (2010). *Welcome to HCUPnet: Statistics on hospital stays.* Retrieved online January 23, 2013, from: http://hcupnet. ahrq.gov.

VBac.com. (2013). *U.S. Cesarean rate dips slightly: Is there hope for more VBACS?* Retrieved online January 23, 2013, from: www.vbac.com/2011/11/u-s-cesarean-rate-dips-slightly-is-there-hope-for-more-vbacs.

Washington, S., Caughey, A. B., Cheng, Y. W., & Bryant, A. S. (2011, September 22). Racial and ethnic differences in indication for primary Cesarean delivery at term: Experience at one U.S. institution. *Birth, 39*(2), 128–134.

Wax, J. R., Cartin, A., Pinette, M. G., & Blackstone, J. (2004) Patient choice Cesarean: An evidence-based review. *Obstetrical and Gynecological Survey, 59,* 601–616.

World Health Organization. (2008a). Appropriate technology for birth. *Lancet,* 2(8452): 436–437.

World Health Organization. (2008b). *Caesarean sections in the world 3: Unnecessary Cesarean sections for year 2008.* Retrieved January 14, 2013, from: www. who.int/entity/healthsystems/topics/financing/healthreport/30C-sectioncosts.pdf.

Wu, J. M., Viswanathan, M., & Ivy, J. S. (2012, November). A conceptual framework for future research on mode of delivery. *Maternal Child Health Journal, 16*, 1447–1454.

Young, D. (2006), "Cesarean Delivery on Maternal Request": Was the NIH Conference Based on a Faulty Premise?. *Birth, 33:* 171–174. doi: 10.1111/j. 1523-536X.2006.00101.x.

Zwelling, E. (2007, June). The emergence of high-tech birthing. *Journal of Obstetrics, Gynecology and Neonatal Nursing, 37*, 85–93. DOI: 10.1111/J.1552-6 909.2007.00211.x.

6 "Hush, Little Baby, Don't Say a Word"

Nursing Narratives through New Media

*Andrée E. C. Betancourt and
Elise E. Labbé*

Story Time, an Opening by Andrée E. C. Betancourt

My 3-year-old son exclaims "Tory Mama, tory Mama, tory Mama!" several times a day, especially before nap and bedtimes, and while using the potty as "the poopsies want to hear the tories too." My 1-year-old son appears to enjoy the stories also and often uses the opportunity to breastfeed in between playing with toys or trying to climb into the bathtub. Along with a hunger for Pedialyte Freezer Pops and my grandmother's empanadas, pregnancy and birth brought cravings for stories about breastfeeding, particularly those traditionally shared as oral histories by women in my family.

My maternal grandmother's body is marked by a story told to her by her mother (Betancourt, 2008). My great-grandmother, a Mexican-Mayan woman, craved cherries when she was pregnant with my grandmother, whom we call Cha. In British Honduras, Cha's native country known today as Belize, cherries were rare. When she was born, Cha brought cherries to her mother in the form of a birthmark on her right arm. When Cha was 8 months old, *un tábano* (a tropical fly) bit the cherries that marked her arm. Her cherries became so infected that the doctors scraped them out of the bone in an attempt to save her arm. Her Belizean father, who had English heritage, donated his much whiter skin from his neck, shoulder, and underarm to restore the place where her cherries had been. The doctor used an electric needle to burn his skin onto her. An aunt, with whom Cha lived in Mexico during her childhood, would put lemon juice in an abalone shell and place it outside to collect the evening dew. Then she would pour it onto my grandmother's arm until it eventually darkened her father's skin, though flecks of white can still be seen. Cha always compares her brown skin to my pale, white skin that erases traces of my Latina heritage. It is through stories such as these that I remain connected to my Mexican-Belizean roots, betrayed by my skin color.

Visits with my mother and maternal grandmother, the two women most central to my upbringing, are limited by the approximately 1000 miles between our homes. Our stories become filtered through mobile phones calls and text messages, email, Facebook, Skype, and Twitter. In the process, the messages become fragmented by dropped calls, weak Internet connections, and computers in need of replacement or upgrades, as well as by my toddler and baby who, fascinated by electronic devices, manage to monopolize, interrupt, and prematurely end conversations.

Introduction and Method

This chapter attempts to voice these fragmented transgenerational connections in ways that engage debates surrounding breastfeeding taboos. It also problematizes the silencing of women whose voices are all too often hushed in the debates because of the taboos surrounding their own experiences of breastfeeding. As Taylor and Wallace (2012) emphasize in their research on breastfeeding and guilt, "as feminist breastfeeding promoters, we must take the lived experiences of mothers as seriously as we take evidence-based biomedical data. ... Only by listening to women can we discover what is important *to them*, what presents challenges *to them*, and what the breastfeeding experience is like *for them*" (p. 201). This chapter foregrounds the limitations and possibilities of new media in the documentation and exchange of breastfeeding experiences, and in doing so, it proposes a model for studying how taboo women's health issues are both voiced and hushed through various mediums.

The challenges of collaboration between a clinical health psychologist (my mother and co-auhtor of this essay Elise) and a communication and media studies scholar (me, Andrée) became apparent early in our research process. Elise, whose research background is primarily quantitative, emailed me: "This type of writing style is hard for me to wrap my head around—but I'm working on it!" Despite differences in our feminist identities, our shared commitment to feminism created a common ground from which we approached our subject matter. As Hausman, Smith, and Labbock (2012) explain in the introduction to their edited collection on breastfeeding, "Standpoint feminism is one approach that seeks to honor women's perspectives on their own experiences. It is a specific version of what Donna Haraway has called *situated knowledge*" (p. 2). Drawing on feminist standpoint theory in an effort to situate ourselves as scholars, mothers who have breastfed multiple children, and in terms of our shared Latina roots and our relationship as mother and daughter, we decided to share our own experiences of breastfeeding.

We are both breastfeeding advocates, yet we ultimately believe that women should do what they believe is best for themselves and their babies. Like Kedrowski and Lipscomb (2008), we share the feminist perspective that "the right to breastfeed, while not absolute and not a duty, is a right that women should fight to win, as part of their broader effort to protect the space of choice that preserves their autonomous control of their bodies—which they give, in numerous ways, to nurture their children" (p. 129). We also found it important to include the experiences of breastfeeding and bottle-feeding shared with us by Cha, the Mexican-Belizean matriarch of our family. Cha's grassroots work with Latina communities on the Gulf Coast, some undocumented and many who struggle to find their voices in English, reminds us of our current privileged positions. Her diverse volunteer work includes performing legal advocacy, teaching English to Spanish speakers, and translating for women during their pre- and postnatal doctor visits. As Calafell and Moreman (2009) assert "While Latinas/os are the largest 'minority' group in the United States, little academic work in the communication field has been attendant to our communities, thus neglecting how these communities are both adding to and changing the academy's theories and practices" (p. 123). This chapter attempts to uncover layers of assimilation that cloud the familial histories that inform our breastfeeding practices as first- and second-generation immigrants.

A Sticky, Leaky Process: Andrée E. C. Betancourt on Navigating Nursing Narratives

Pleased with the content Elise generated on psychological research on our two primary topics, breastfeeding and social media, I was troubled by her distant, self-conscious narrative about breastfeeding experiences that she shared with me through email. It did not produce the rhythm of her voice or intimate details that usually appear in her stories. She took a removed social scientist approach, and it is apparent that she was voicing a story to an audience of strangers. As co-authors, we are not afforded the anonymity granted to interview subjects. We strive for openness in an effort to confront taboos, but our negotiation of professional and familial identities results in many things left unsaid. My mother and grandmother's pro-breastfeeding narratives struck me as romanticized as I began my fourth year of breastfeeding on demand, a joyful yet tedious labor of love. Nadesan and Sotirin (1998) offer a description of breastfeeding "as a form of mediating sensuality" in an effort to "promote an alternative articulation of, and performative possibilities for, the breast-feeding mother (and child)." Nadesan and Sotorin's approach problematizes the dualism created by the use of the discursive complexes "the romance of the natural mother" and "the science of breast-feeding" in the advocacy of the "breast is best" claim (p. 229). My maternal body experiences the "polymorphous sensations" that Nadesan and Sotirin articulate as pleasures such as "multiple points of bodily contact, moments of caress, enveloping feelings of well-being, and warmth stimulated by the chemical process in lactation," along with the pains "of milk production in the breast (letdown, engorgement, etc.), bodily fatigue and aches, and the pain of scratches, kicks, and bites." My baby and I perhaps even realize the possibility of "synchronicity of corporeal sensations that constitute a dialogic mutuality of bodies" (p. 229).

Some of the bruises from my baby's pinching and kneading of my body as he nurses are visible around the necklines of my clothes, and my mother lays her hands on me gently with concern. She is the only one who can tell me how I nursed as a baby, and she assures me that I did not perform wild acrobatics like my sons do when they breastfeed—though she notes that one of my brothers did. As Case (2009) reminds us in her performance about cancer stories, "we *all* fail to represent ourselves accurately, and our own narrations of our own histories can't ever be complete. *None* of us narrates alone; we *must* rely on others to help us each make sense of our own memories and histories" (p. 258). I was 16 when my youngest brother was born, but I have no clear memories of my mother breastfeeding my four younger siblings. I do, however, have vague memories of her using breast pads. Breastfeeding memories, like the process of nursing, can be leaky, and through sharing them we must negotiate various types of exposure that violate cultural norms.

This chapter maps out how my mother and grandmother's shared experiences of breastfeeding travel through me as lead author and what happens to my story in the process. The following section frames our entry to this project as independent scholar and professor, respectively. It is followed by a review of recent, primarily quantitative, research on breastfeeding and social media; Labbé's breastfeeding narrative and Betancourt's questioning of what is left unvoiced; Betancourt's interviews with her Mexican-Belizean grandmother; and a conclusion that suggests directions for future research.

Breastfeeding as an Ivory Tower Taboo: Andrée E. C. Betancourt's Breastfeeding Narrative

As a mother in the academic job market, writing this chapter is in itself a taboo act. I hesitate to list it on my curriculum vitae. Although prospective employers should not discriminate against those who breastfeed or write scholarly articles about breastfeeding, it is no secret that some do. At a job fair held during a convention in my field, I was keenly aware of the gawking my pregnant body received from many of the departmental representatives staffing booths. Their avoidance of eye contact through sudden immersion in a conversation with someone else or through preoccupation with the arrangement of brochures, was quite different from the reception I received at job fairs at this convention during previous years when I was not pregnant. In their book on academic motherhood, Connelly and Ghodsee (2011) state that "the academic studies of the effect of parenthood and the academy do show a negative correlation between parenthood and tenure for women" (p. 13). They reference Mason and Goulden's 2002–2003 study of ladder-rank faculty at the nine University of California campuses that found that a woman in academia "was more likely to be single, more likely to be divorced, and more likely to delay childbearing, potentially until it is too late" (p. 15). They note Mason and Goulden's study reveals that "whereas only 20 percent of men claimed that they had fewer children than they wanted, the percentage points were twice as high for women" (p. 15). The majority of our female academic colleagues are childless or have only one or two children, similar to the rates reported in a 2002 study that found female professors had an average of .66 children each in comparison to the national average of two children (Wilson, 2009, p. 18).

In response to a professor friend of mine posting a link on Facebook to the article, "The Case Against Breast-feeding" (Rosin, 2009), the daughter of a female academic commented: "As a 29-year-old feminist academic who might someday be a mom, I'm really worried. If the mothers I see around me who share my race and socioeconomic class, and even my profession, are too stressed and overwhelmed to breastfeed, do I really want to have a child?" My professor friend replied, "Your first comment breaks my heart. Every mama that wrote a comment (including me) feeds her kid breastmilk—the only academic mamas that don't that I know are ones who adopt. (the nonacademics drop before six months unless they are stay-at-home moms because breastfeeding, as Sears says, is a 'lifestyle') ... there's much more to raising a child than breastmilk." The mixed messages about motherhood and breastfeeding in academia can be distressing. Fighting tears as she walked to teach her first course as a new mother "with breasts full with milk that (her) daughter would not drink until later," Hudock (2008) asserts that "to enter a university classroom, I know that I must perform childlessness, like I perform the characteristics of my gender, my class, my ethnicity, my education" (pp. 63–64). Even more disturbing than mixed messages is the silence on the topic, especially when it involves advisors who may have experienced at first hand the repercussions of motherhood on their academic careers and yet are unwilling or feel unable to voice their experiences to those they mentor.

As a childless graduate student participant of the 2007 NCA Convention, I attended a panel on motherhood. I did not know any of the other attendees, who I remember as being female. Tucked away at the end of a hallway, I felt that it was a secretive gathering. After all, why would anyone wish to associate herself openly with motherhood in an academic setting when doing so is risky? Deanna Shoemaker's (2011) performance of "Mamafesto! Why Superheroes Wear Capes" stuck with me, especially years later as I grappled with the tensions of new motherhood and academia. Shoemaker's repetitive singing of lyrics from Woody Guthrie's song "'I'll Eat You, I'll Drink You" is what I remembered most vividly of her performance as I struggled with fervently nursing my five weeks premature son in an effort to raise his low birth weight and discontinue the supplementation of formula ordered by our midwives and pediatrician. I did not remember all of the words that Shoemaker sang, but I knew that they captured the conflicting feelings of being exhaustingly consumed around the clock by a tiny, precious human. Bits from the chorus Shoemaker sang surfaced as memories of consuming her, a stranger who shared secrets with others hungry for bits of motherhood at a convention whose conventions keep motherhood invisible, sustained me: "I'm a-gonna eat you up. I'm gonna drink you down" (p. 192).

At times brutally painful, the experience of breastfeeding was also magical in terms of being physically connected to my delicious newborn in a manner that nourished him in countless ways. I sang to my baby what I remembered of the song "Cowgirl in the Sand," by Neil Young that my mother sang to my siblings and me as she nursed us, and the "Sapito" lullaby that my grandmother sang to us in Spanish, while my mom, who birthed me when she was an undergraduate student, was studying or working. When not trying every trick in the book to keep my baby awake long enough to nurse (he did not have the strength to keep himself awake for feedings), I was attached to a monstrous aquamarine colored breast pump that we rented from the birth center in an effort to keep my milk supply up. Shoemaker (2011), who composed bits and pieces of "Mamafesto" while performing other acts such as breastfeeding, explains that it "aspires to open up spaces of dialogue about the complex and sometimes impossible 'balancing acts' required of mothers who work full-time, as well as to manifest institutional changes for caregivers and academics more broadly" (p. 191). Often ravenous after nursing and pumping so frequently, but too weak and tired to prepare meals, I nursed myself with nutrition shakes.

I detest having to use a breast pump instead of nursing my babies in person, and I suspect that if I worked full-time outside the home I would not be breastfeeding as long. The results of a study of the impact of workplace practices on breastfeeding "suggest that maternal access to their babies and structural support for breastfeeding in the workplace are the most important factors affecting women's ability to continue breastfeeding after resuming employment" (Lubold & Roth, 2012, p. 164). I turn to Facebook for clues on how new mothers in academia today negotiate breastfeeding.[1] One professor friend posted this status update: "getting ready for the semester: made a pumping sign for my office door. i've never seen one before, so here's hoping it does the trick ..." along with an image of the sign that reads "My mama is pumping. Please do not disturb. Thank you!" Signed with her son's name, it features a photograph of him drinking from a bottle. Her post is followed by 15 comments, including her update "the head of my area decided to hold the first meeting of my area during the only time i have to pump tomorrow in our all-day grad orientation extravanganza (and, no, he would not be comfortable with me pumping at the meeting—and given who is there, i probably wouldn't be either). so, the sign comes out of me deciding that that i can't be ashamed of making feeding my child a priority in my life right now. so, i *really* appreciate all the love and support here!!" This update was followed by supportive comments, and several female friends wrote that they were motivated to make nursing signs or improve their current ones.

A freelance assignment shortly after my first son's birth required that I work 60 hours one week. My breast pump was inspected by the client's security guards after passing through the X-ray scanner; thankfully, this was before my spouse had to repair it using duct tape and chop sticks in an effort to make it work properly after my toddler dropped it. The client, a federal government agency, would probably have provided a place for me to pump. However, as a contractor I did not want to mark myself as a new mother and risk discrimination, so I endured pumping my breasts in the bathroom. Turning to Twitter, I find a number of tweets that echo challenges and concerns women face pumping at their workplaces such as: "Baby isnt even here yet and I'm terrified to go back to work bc I know they're going to give me hell about breastfeeding and pumping" (Kayyslayy, 2013) and "Work with a bunch of guys. Wonder what they thought when the saw the breast pump sterilization kit in the microwave at lunch" (MarcialEva, 2013). The steady lullaby of breastfeeding-related tweets increased in volume significantly over the controversy surrounding American University professor Adrienne Pine who brought her sick baby to her feminist anthropology course and briefly breastfed her while carrying on her lecture.

Like Deanna Shoemaker, who performs warnings from colleagues that foreground her research on motherhood as "dangerous" to her academic career, Alison Bartlett (2005) highlights the taboos surrounding breastfeeding by describing her closeted research process that led to her book *Breastwork*. Bartlett embarked upon the project in response to being "appalled" by most of the breastfeeding literature she read, particularly work that featured a "very moralistic and prescriptive tone" (p. 2). She confesses:

> I did this secretly, as I was supposed to be working on an Australian writer whose gender was rather fluid and ambiguous. But I was immersed in a new and decidedly gendered role of mothering and found that I needed to make sense of my own changed subjectivity. ... I regarded the breastfeeding article I wrote as a rider to my proper work, a temporary tangent that would pass, just as I imagined breastfeeding would soon pass from my life. But neither did. (pp. 2–3)

Finding limitations in dualistic conceptualizations of breastfeeding to be "natural," Bartlett draws on Judith Butler's (2006) early notion of the performative in her argument that "breastfeeding can more productively be read as performative: as an act that we do, either consciously, or unconsciously, as part of our cultural negotiation of gender" (p. 5). Building upon Bartlett's work, this chapter also engages performances of breastfeeding as a cultural practice: our own performances, as well as those we have witnessed personally or learned of through shared narratives.

Just the Facts: Setting the Stage

Breastfeeding and Social Media

Todd Wolynn (2012), the chief executive officer for the National Breastfeeding Center, calls for using social media to inform, encourage, and support women who are considering breastfeeding or who are breastfeeding. He argues that these young women view information from social media as trusted "'friends'—not just as we traditionally define them, but also as they have redefined them: as the people and organizations within their online social media networks" (p. 364). Healthcare organizations are beginning to realize the potential usefulness of social media as a means of improving patients' responses to medical intervention as well as promoting healthy behaviors (Robledo, 2012). Robledo proposes a three-pronged approach to integrating social media for health communication in an obstetrics and gynecology specialty of high-risk maternal health. He recommends that independent sources of content such as Twitter, Facebook, health data tracking tools, and contact information be integrated into mobile applications. This allows input from patients as well as the ability to evaluate whether the social media and other types of content are actually helpful to the users. It also permits mothers to receive more personalized messages and feedback about their health and health behavior. In reviewing the few research studies specifically on breastfeeding and social media, little empirical data is available to determine the effects of social media on taboos about breastfeeding.

Biopsychosocial Effects of Breastfeeding

The research on the biopsychosocial effects of breastfeeding on mother and infant over the past few decades clearly indicates that breastfeeding is beneficial for the infant in all areas of functioning, including emotional regulation and overall health (Smith & Ellwood, 2011; Wolynn, 2012). For example, children who are exclusively breastfed tend to show significant and positive differences in verbal IQ scores, compared to mixed-fed infants and only formula-fed infants (Kramer et al., 2008). In another example, research results indicated that children who were exclusively breastfed were less likely to experience respiratory or ear infections compared to those experiencing other feeding combinations (Hetzner, Razza, Malone, & Brooks-Gunn, 2009). Although other studies have found that mixed-fed babies also fare significantly better in all areas of biopsychosocial functioning than formula-only fed babies (Kramer et al., 2008).

Smith and Ellwood (2011) were interested in trying to determine the mechanisms that might account for the positive psychosocial effects of breastfeeding on mothers. They tracked mothers at 3, 6, and 9 months postpartum using a time survey record of infant feeding for 24 hours for 7 days using an electronic device. Their findings suggest that time spent in emotional care was positively correlated with time spent breastfeeding. Emotional care included activities such as soothing, holding, or cuddling the infant. Infants that were exclusively breastfed received the greatest amount of emotional care from their mothers. Mixed-fed babies received more emotional care than formula-fed infants but not as much as exclusively breastfed infants. Smith and Ellwood (2011) propose that this greater emotional care may have a positive impact on cognitive development. More research needs to be conducted to obtain a better understanding of the mechanisms that create the positive effects of breastfeeding on infants' cognitive development.

Although there is relatively good research indicating the positive effects of breastfeeding on infant and maternal health, the effects of breastfeeding on the mother–child bond have also been studied. A review of the research on breastfeeding and the mother–infant relationship found scant evidence for clear positive effects (Jansen, de Weerth, & Riksen-Walraven, 2008). Jansen et al. found that theoretical mechanisms described in both human and animal models propose the benefits of breastfeeding on the maternal bond. However, the few empirical studies the researchers found do not provide strong evidence one way or the other. Thus, Jansen et al. propose that the decision to breastfeed should not be made for this reason alone.

There has also been interest in determining what factors might increase the likelihood of mothers breastfeeding their infant. In one qualitative study of 25 Midwestern women who were breastfeeding their infants, researchers found that some psychosocial factors might influence the decision for mothers to exclusively breastfeed (Bai, Middlestadt, Peng, & Fly, 2009). Mothers reported that breastfeeding helped them bond with their babies and that it would make their babies healthier. They were more likely to note that family and friends approved of their breastfeeding but that people in public places generally did not. McMillan et al. (2008) evaluated the effectiveness of the theory of planned behavior and other psychological variables in predicting whether mothers would choose to breastfeed their infants. They sampled 248 women while they were still in the hospital, at discharge, and 10 days and 6 weeks postpartum. The results indicated that certain attitudes and beliefs, especially those related to moral norm, predicted both intention and breastfeeding behavior across time. Moral norm in the theory of planned behavior refers to a person's feeling that he or she should or should not engage in a certain behavior (Ajzen, 1991). If the women did not respond according to their moral norm, they would feel guilty; or they would feel right if they behaved in accordance to the moral norm. This finding is relevant in terms of how social media can influence a person's moral norm and encourage or discourage taboos regarding breastfeeding. However, the research on the effects of social media on taboos about breastfeeding is scant and so does not permit evaluation.

Between the Lines

Elise E. Labbé's Breastfeeding Narrative

I didn't have a mobile phone, Internet access, or Facebook when I was breastfeeding my five children through my 20s and 30s. I did seek out information through books and from my mother-in-law who had breastfed all of her 11 children. I clearly remember her coming to the hospital and giving me a mini-lesson on breastfeeding. At that time, no one in the healthcare system gave me any information about the importance of breastfeeding and how to pull it off successfully. I also remember that she had made some kind of instant tea mix with Nestea iced tea and orange mix. She encouraged me to mix up a hot cup of it and drink it while I breastfed. It was supposed to help me relax and encourage the milk flow—it seemed to work well! She is now in her 80s, and when I asked her about the tea drink so that I could make some for my daughter and daughter-in-law for when they breastfeed, she couldn't remember.

Although breastfeeding wasn't encouraged when I gave birth to my first baby, I didn't experience any social pressure not to. Maybe because it was in the 1970s in New Orleans and people there tended to be in a "live and let live" mode. I did find it challenging at times to comfortably nurse in public places, and I frequently found myself being embarrassed when my breasts would leak all over. We didn't have all the great contraptions we have today, especially those high-powered breast pumps. I remember trying to hand pump and giving up on it. Since I went back to college classes, and later work, for all of my children within a week or two of giving birth, I would have to run home at lunchtime and in the afternoon to feed them. I was okay with my spouse and caretakers giving them formula if I couldn't make it in time. By taking a "flow as you go" approach, I was able to breastfeed most of my children until they were 2 years old.

Although breastfeeding was sometimes a hassle, it really was an efficient and financially more effective way to feed my children. I loved the experience of holding them close, looking into their beautiful and loving eyes and being still with them. I believe breastfeeding strengthened my bond with my children and contributed to them being healthy children. I also believe my Hispanic roots, from my mother's side, influenced my positive attitude about breastfeeding. Experiencing touch, being comfortable with my body, especially the sexual nature of being a woman, and creating strong mother–child bonds were encouraged by my Hispanic mother as well as by my aunts and uncles.

A Daughter Hungry for More: Andrée E. C. Betancourt's Response

As part of our research process, we created a closed Facebook group called Breastfeeding and Social Media and invited Friends to post their own experiences. A cousin on my father's side of the family wrote to my mother "Elise, you were one of the first women I knew in my generation who breastfed, … I recall sitting with you in a bedroom talking about it while you were nursing [your son] at the family Christmas party at my mother's house on Argonne, and how calm you were about it. Had a big influence on me as I didn't have kids yet." After reading Elise's narrative, I note that she avoided topics that would have addressed some of the hardships she faced such as breastfeeding as a low-income student and as a single mother to three children and living 1000 miles away from family. I find a few more clues about my mother's breastfeeding experience in a booklet (Ochsner Clinic Department of Pediatrics) that she received from the hospital after I was born. She crossed out two sentences—one that suggested making babies go for four hours between feedings, and the other recommending not giving bottles to breastfed babies, with the possible exception of one time per night if it is "the only way" for the mother to get sleep (p. 12). The booklet is pro-breastfeeding, yet the majority of the content is about bottle-feeding. It assures new mothers that their bottle-fed babies will be "just as healthy" as breastfed ones, and asserts: "Modern formulas are as good as breast milk, but you will be missing something—most mothers find nursing a rather special experience" (p. 18).

Milky Memories: From Belize to the Gulf Coast

A Late Night Feeding

In the introduction to her study of performing birth stories that "resist shame and silence, at least in part, by throwing off narrative norms," Della Pollock (2006) recounts asking her mother for her birth story: "She tried to accommodate my interest. ... Her story, like what we typically think of as a good story, had a beginning and end, but no middle. She was "knocked out" for the delivery, eager but able only to construct a story out of narrative tropes and the logic of efficiency/outcomes. What loomed in the middle silence was the unspoken because unquestioned authority of medical science" (p. 7). Like Pollock's mother, my grandmother was also "'knocked out'" for the births of both of her daughters. Although the "twilight sleep" erased her memories of the births, she has not forgotten her short-lived breast-feeding experience and the faulty medical science that led her to bottle-feed her daughters. My grandmother, Barbara Martha Labbé, known to most as Cha, immigrated from Belize City to New Orleans in 1953 alone at the age of 20. She shared her breastfeeding experience with me in person late one night in December 2012.

ANDRÉE: Did your mother breastfeed you?

CHA: All of us were breastfed. She would sneak off early so she could go to church. She would leave all of her clothes downstairs for mass on Sunday morning, but if [my father] realized she was up and getting ready he would make noise so the baby would wake. He wasn't Catholic. He didn't go to mass. He was Church of England. ... He would make noise so baby would wake up and have to be breastfed and not go to church.

ANDRÉE: Breastfeeding was what people did?

CHA: Definitely. We didn't have the modern conveniences ... bottles. You were criticized if you didn't breastfeed. People would think that you didn't want to have the child. I didn't think it was as prominent here. In the States I never saw anyone breastfeeding, actually.

ANDRÉE: When you became a mother were people breastfeeding?

CHA: Not as much I don't think. Not as much.

ANDRÉE: Did you breastfeed my mother?

CHA: I must have breastfed her till she was about 8 weeks old, and see let me explain. I was supposed to go back for my post-delivery checkup. Like six weeks afterwards and my doctor was out of town. The lady said I could see his partner but I didn't like him. When he got back he examined me and said that he wanted me to go to the hospital immediately as when I had Elise I had heavy bleeding and they had to close me up quickly. Unknown to me I was diagnosed as a GI (gastrointestinal) bleeder and I guess that's what made me bleed so much but I don't know how we could find out today as things have changed so much. I was on the verge of having peritonitis, a serious infection. They didn't get rid of all of the afterbirth. Before I left the hospital they told me that I would probably not be able to breastfeed Elise because of the shock to my body and the next morning sure enough my milk was dried up. I told the doctor that can't go now because I have an eight-week-old baby and my mother is taking care of her so I have to make arrangements. He would only let me go if I promised to come back. I went home and got Elise situated, and my husband admitted me. So they dilated me and they went in and cleaned out. I had your mom then I had [your aunt] and everything went well. When I was pregnant with Elise they thought I was going to lose her so they gave me some shots. They were the safe ones as I had no reactions and both of my daughters were born good. Now we know that's not true. If I had had a way to stimulate my breast the milk would have come back.

ANDRÉE: What did my mother drink?

CHA: Similac. I think it was Enfamil or Similac. I think we had both of them. They both were on the market but check that out. And by the time she was 8 months old I was feeding her table food.

ANDRÉE: How did you feel about all of that?

CHA: Truthfully, it didn't bother me as I was in the hands of a good doctor, and I knew that he was treating me, and I never thought of it as something that would damage Elise. In Belize, if you couldn't breastfeed children were raised on artificial powered milk called Klim. It spelled milk backward. It came from England. I think it's because the way we were raised. You just followed your physician's advice ... it wasn't until my daughters grew up and told me I could have stimulated the mammary glands ... by suckling or palpating or whatever they call that. And I never thought that not having the breast milk would hinder her growth. She was growing fine and was a healthy child.

As the interview continued, my grandmother began telling me about what would be considered taboo family history related to my own childhood. Although she knew I was doing research on breastfeeding, the questions that I asked about her and my great-grandmother's experience breastfeeding provoked answers that also dealt with other topics such as religion, education, and abuse. She became caught up in unexpected memories and shared these with me. Knowing how foreign the Belize and Mexico of her youth are to her US-born family members, in sharing her past, Cha always provides us with great detail. Before I could ask her questions about breastfeeding her second child, my second child woke up to nurse and our interview was cut short. My son's hunger trumped my appetite for my grandmother's memories, so I gave her *un beso* goodnight and then rushed to answer his call.

Continuing Through Skype

Separated again by many miles, we used Skype for a second interview in February 2013. Diagnosed with cancer, follicular lymphoma, in August 2012, Cha lost hair during chemotherapy and was wearing a headscarf.

ANDRÉE: Did you breastfeed your second daughter?

CHA: After she was born, there was no milk at all so I might have breastfed her a little, but I gave her formula as I never really got a lot of milk.

ANDRÉE: Were other people you knew breastfeeding?

CHA: Several of my neighbors were breastfeeding.

ANDRÉE: Did the doctor say anything about you not being able to breastfeed?

CHA: No. Never said a thing. Just went on like it was the natural thing. No one ever said anything or tried to convince me.

ANDRÉE: Did your mother say anything to you about breastfeeding?

CHA: My mother had breastfed years ago, at least 9 years ago. It was like [breastfeeding] was over. There is nothing to worry about it.

ANDRÉE: How did you feel about it?

CHA: I can't even think about it right now, like if it made an impression on me. I just took it like: that's how it going to be.

ANDRÉE: Did you think it was related to your doctor telling you that you weren't going to be able to nurse your first daughter?

CHA: Yes, I do believe that I thought that's what it was. I think that somewhere along the way the doctor told me that I would never be able to breastfeed again.

ANDRÉE: What did you think about your first daughter breastfeeding her children?

CHA: I thought it was wonderful. I thought that it was very fortunate that she could do it. I heard how well it makes you look, and I was convinced that it was part of her getting back into shape.

ANDRÉE: What did you think about your second daughter breastfeeding her children?

CHA: I don't think she breastfed as long as your mom, but I was happy that it looked to me like she could do it.

ANDRÉE: You mentioned in December that you never saw anyone in the US breastfeeding, did you see the neighbors who you mentioned breastfeeding?

CHA: Yes, but it was not awkward, and only inside. You hardly ever saw anyone breastfeeding like you girls do.

Cha had her babies in the late 1950s, around the time when pregnancy had become increasingly medicalized in a manner that promoted infant formula for being "scientifically" designed and manufactured, whereas breast milk "was seen as inferior, possibly unsanitary, and difficult to measure" (Kedrowski & Lipscomb, 2008, p. 6). Labbock (2012) explains that

> [t]he practice of formula feeding was bolstered by a call for women in the workplace during World War II, a women's movement largely centered on worksite equity and reproductive freedom, and an onslaught of advertising by formula companies reassuring them by emphasizing that formula-feeding is safe, clean, neat, easy, and a modern "mother's helper." Hence, women came to understand breastfeeding as unsafe, dirty, messy, difficult, antiquated, and antiwoman. (p. 39)

The frustration of not having been breastfed due to the misinformation my grandmother received motivated my mother and her sister to nurse their own children. My aunt was fired from her elementary school teaching position in the 1980s for being pregnant; the religious school where she taught was uncomfortable with pregnant and lactating bodies in the classroom—a sentiment still echoed by some today. As part of her argument for a rights-framework versus a choice-framework for breastfeeding, Hausman (2012) argues that "Dominant ideologies focus women's attention on their own bodies as lacking rather than on social systems that fail to support their practices and goals" (p. 18). Noting that "inadequate milk supply is the most common reason given for early weaning," Hausman asserts: "Women perceive low milk supply to be a biological failure of their bodies, yet it is most often the effect of poor lactation management, which is itself a social constraint in a cultural context unfamiliar with the demands of breastfeeding" (p. 18). Despite not being able to breastfeed, Taylor and Wallace (2012) found that the term *shame*, as opposed to the term *guilt*, more accurately describes the dominant feeling that women express about formula feeding (p. 193). Cha voiced neither guilt nor shame over formula-feeding, yet upon reflection realized that medical authorities undermined her maternal authority.

Conclusion

Elise E. Labbé on Social Media, Mothering, and Mindfulness

In working with Andrée on this chapter, I found myself becoming more aware of how social media are having a major impact on health communication and that this impact can have positive as well as negative effects. I asked my youngest daughter—a 22-year-old member of Generation Y—if she would consider using Twitter to express how she felt about breastfeeding. She was horrified by the idea and said she would get grief from friends wondering why she would tweet about breastfeeding if she is not pregnant or currently considering pregnancy. Interestingly enough, she is supportive of a best friend who has been breastfeeding for a year. Therefore, it seems that just discussing some types of topics using social media might be taboo in and of itself. As I engage more heavily in social media, keeping up with friends and family, I become overwhelmed with the energy and time it takes to "plug in." However, the new media are often the most practical way to stay in touch with my adult children. Although breastfeeding my babies seemed to be time efficient and provided me with quiet time for myself and my children, I wonder if mothers today experience nursing as taking time away from their social media time. I noted that Andrée often has her iPad and iPhone nearby when she starts breastfeeding. Might using social media while breastfeeding reduce some of the emotional positive effects that I experienced as a mother who breastfed "unplugged?"

When breastfeeding, a mother might use that time to be mindful of what she is doing with her infant, thus allowing her to be present in the moment with her baby. Mindfulness is attending to the present moment with openness, nonjudging, nonstriving, acceptance, patience, trust, and letting go (Labbé, 2011). Fostering mindfulness can decrease the negative reactions a mother might have about some aspects of breastfeeding and at the same time create gratefulness and loving-kindness. Research on mindfulness indicates that higher levels of mindfulness are associated with resilience and better emotional regulation (Labbé, Womble, & Shenesey, 2011). By taking a few relaxing breaths before nursing and bringing one's attention to the infant and self, a mother can learn to let go of tension and stress. This in turn can help the infant relax and foster a loving bond between mother and child.

From an empirical standpoint, there is much that we do not know about the effects of social media on women's choice to breastfeed as well as the potential for the creation or abandonment of taboos related to breastfeeding. There is good evidence that breastfeeding has positive biopsychosocial effects for both mother and infant. We do not have a lot of information available for the mechanisms underlying some of these positive outcomes. Our research process confirmed my belief that breastfeeding your infant is a good thing to do for a variety of reasons. However, forcing or criticizing a mother for not choosing to breastfeed might negate some of the positive effects of breastfeeding. Social media can be used to provide data to those who are considering breastfeeding so that they can make an informed decision. Presentation of that data will be more impactful if it is communicated at a personal level and from "trusted" social media friends.

Andrée E. C. Betancourt on Breastfeeding in Belize
and the Digital Divide

In her performance about cancer stories, Case (2009) asserts that "[t]here's a very fine line between *telling* someone's story and *taking* someone's story, but it's a line worth walking. Stories can't be separated from one another. You can't tell your own story without telling someone else's. Stories don't begin, and they don't end. You can only start and stop a story, and save some parts for later" (p. 258). In working with Elise on this chapter, I experienced the challenge of untangling various versions of the "same" family stories that are voiced differently by generation, geographic location, and through the use of new media. According to the Centers for Disease Control and Prevention (2015), the National Immunization Survey (NIS) found that the percentage of babies, born between 2009 and 2012, who are breastfed has increased. The NIS estimates that 80.0±1.2 of U.S. babies, born in 2012, were breastfed (Percentage ± half 95% Confidence Interval). The percentages in these surveys deceased to 51.4±1.5 at 6 months, and 29.2±1.4 at 12 months for babies born in 2012. In comparison, of the babies born in 2009 included in the surveys: 76.1±1.0 were breastfed; 46.6±1.2 at 6 months, and 24.6±1.0 at 12 months. The percentages were lower for babies exclusively breastfed for 6 months, though these rates have also been increasing: from 15.6±0.9 for babies born in 2009 to 21.9±1.4 for babies born in 2012. Leah Bennett (2013) reports that "[a]mong Belize's diverse population, those least likely to breastfeed exclusively for the crucial first three months were better-educated women, mostly from urban areas and with careers, and within the Creole community, the country's ministry reports. The highest rate of exclusive breastfeeding was among the Q'eqch'i Maya and women who gave birth at home." Although it appears that breastfeeding rates will continue to increase in both the United States and Belize (Bennett, 2013), as Hausman, Smith and Labbok (2012) argue, it remains problematic that breastfeeding is blamed "as a source of women's inequality" when the blame should actually be placed on "the political, economic, and sociocultural constraints in women's lives that make breastfeeding difficult" (p. 3).

A younger family friend from Belize who was not breastfed, possibly because her older sister had an allergic reaction to breast milk, responded to me through Facebook about contemporary attitudes about breastfeeding. Her Spanish mother-in-law did not breastfeed because of the lower-class stigma her generation associated with the act. My friend and her sister remember the Breast Is Best League campaign founded in 1981 in Belize, which, according to a 1987 report, was a model program and none other existed in the Caribbean at the time. Despite the challenge posed by inverted nipples, her sister breastfed using pumped milk. After learning more about the benefits from peers in Spain, my Belizean friend plans to breastfeed if she has children, but believes that it is unpopular in Belize because of "the effort, time, and work" involved.

Belizeans have significantly less Internet access than individuals in the United States: 26.77% of the population versus 86.75% as of July 2014 (Internet Live Stats, 2014). Social media, therefore, is not as accessible to new mothers in Belize who might use it as a resource if considering breastfeeding. Further research is needed to examine the effects of the digital divide on Belizean mothers' baby feeding decisions and experiences. For some parents with Internet access, social media replace or extend the use of traditional baby books in the recording of both mundane moments and milestones in their children's lives. I used Facebook to share the experience of my toddler attempting to breastfeed his baby brother, and perhaps future generations will "like" and "comment" upon that status update. Social media is likely to have an increasingly important role in linking shared memories of the ways in which we were first nourished and in the mapping of challenges that women face in voicing their baby feeding experiences.

Note

1. We have intentionally not corrected spelling or grammar of content quoted from sources such as Facebook status updates and Tweets.

References

Ajzen, I. (1991). The theory of planned behavior. *Organizational Behavior and Human Decision Processes, 50*, 179–211.

Bai, Y. K., Middlestadt, S. E., Peng, C.-Y, & Fly, A. D. (2009). Psychosocial factors underlying the mother's decision to continue exclusive breastfeeding for 6 months: An elicitation study. *Journal of Human Nutrition and Dietetics, 22*, 134–140. DOI:10.1111/j.1365-277X.2009.00950.x.

Bartlett, A. (2005). *Breastwork: Rethinking breastfeeding.* Sydney, NSW: University of New South Wales Press.

Betancourt, A. (Director). (2008, November 21). *Agridulce.* Performed at the National Communication Association Convention, Hilton San Diego Bayfront, San Diego, CA.

Butler, J. (2006). *Gender trouble: Feminism and the subversion of identity.* New York: Routledge.

Calafell, B. M., & Moreman, S. T. (2009). Envisioning an academic readership: Latina/o performativities per the form of publication. *Text and Performance Quarterly, 29*, 123–130.

Case, G. (2009). Apoptosis is my favorite word: An introduction and performance. *Literature and Medicine, 28*(2), 253–272. Retrieved February 20, 2013, from Project MUSE database.

Centers for Disease Control and Prevention. (2015, July 31). Breastfeeding among U.S. children born 2002–2012, CDC National Immunization Surveys. Retrieved October 7, 2015, from http://www.cdc.gov/breastfeeding/data/nis_data/index.htm.

Connelly, R., & Ghodsee, K. (2011). *Professor mommy: Finding work-family balance in academia.* Lanham, MD: Rowman & Littlefield.

Davanzo, R., Zauli, G., Monasta, L., Brumatti, L. V., Abate, M. V., Ventura, G., et al. (2012). Human colostrum and breast milk contain high levels of

TNF-related apoptosis-inducing ligand (TRAIL). *Journal of Human Lactation,* 29(1), 23–25.

Hausman, B. L. (2012). Feminism and breastfeeding: Rhetoric, ideology, and the material realities of women's lives. In P. H. Smith, B. L. Hausman, & M. Labbock (Eds.), *Beyond health, beyond choice: breastfeeding constraints and realities* (pp. 15–24). New Brunswick, NJ: Rutgers University Press.

Hausman, B. L., Smith, P. H., & Labbock, M. (2012). Introduction: Breastfeeding constraints and realties. In P. H. Smith, B. L. Hausman, & M. Labbock (Eds.), *Beyond health, beyond choice: Breastfeeding constraints and realities* (pp. 1–11). New Brunswick, NJ: Rutgers University Press.

Hetzner, N. M. P., Razza, R. A., Malone, L. M., & Brooks-Gunn, J. (2009). Associations among feeding behaviors during infancy and child illness at two years. *Maternal and Child Health Journal, 13,* 795–805.

Hudock, A. (2008). First day of school. In E. Evans & C. Grant (Eds.), *Mama, PhD: Women write about motherhood and academic life* (pp. 63–65). Piscataway, NJ: Rutgers University Press.

Internet Live Stats. (2014). Internet users by country (2014). Retrieved October 7, 2015, from http://www.internetlivestats.com/internet-users-by-country/.

Jansen, J., de Weerth, C., & Riksen-Walraven, J. M. (2008). Breastfeeding and the mother infant relationship—A review. *Developmental Review, 28,* 503–521.

Kayyslayy. (2013, January 25). [Twitter post.] Retrieved from https://twitter.com/kayyslayy/status/294739136898797568.

Kedrowski, K. M., & Lipscomb, M. E. (2008). *Breastfeeding rights in the United States.* Westport, CT: Praeger.

Kramer, M. S., Aboud, F., Mironova, E., Vanilovich, I., Platt, R. W., Matush, L., et al. (2008). Promotion of breastfeeding intervention trial (PROBIT) study group. *Archives of General Psychiatry, 65,* 578–584. doi:10.1001/archpsyc.65.5.578.

Labbock, M. (2012). Breastfeeding in public health: What is needed for policy and program action? In Smith, P. H., Hausman, B. L., & Labbock, M. (Eds.), *Beyond health, beyond choice: Breastfeeding constraints and realities* (pp. 36–50). New Brunswick, NJ: Rutgers University Press.

Labbé, E. (2011). *Psychology moment by moment: A guide to enhancing your clinical practice with mindfulness and meditation.* Oakland, CA: New Harbinger.

Labbé, E. E., Womble, M., & Shenesey, J. (2011). Exploring the relationship between mindfulness and resilience. In C. A. Stark & D. C. Bonner (Eds.), *Handbook on spirituality: Belief systems, societal impact and roles in coping* (pp. 303–312). Hauppauge, NY: Nova Science.

Lubold, A. M., & Roth, L. M. (2012). The impact of workplace practices on breastfeeding experiences and disparities among women. In Smith, P. H., Hausman, B. L., & Labbock, M. (Eds.), *Beyond health, beyond choice: Breastfeeding constraints and realities* (pp. 157–166). New Brunswick, NJ: Rutgers University Press.

MarcialEva. (2013, January 20). [Twitter post.] Retrieved from https://twitter.com/MarcialEva/status/293214589905162240.

Mason, A. M., & Goulden, M. (2004). Marriage and baby blues: Redefining gender equity in the academy. Annals of the American Academy of Political and Social Science, 596, 86–103.

McMillan, B., Conner, M., Woolridge, M., Dyson, L., Green, J., Renfrew, M., et al. (2008). Predicting breastfeeding in women living in areas of economic hardship: Explanatory role of the theory of planned behavior. *Psychology and Health, 23,* 767–788.

Mjrobbins. (2009, May 29). [Twitter post.] Retrieved from https://twitter.com/mjrobbins/status/1960646796.

Mohamad, E. (2012). Breasts, bags, clothes and shoes: Constructing motherhood and images of breastfeeding vs. formula feeding women. *Asian Social Science, 8,* 93–106. doi: 10.5539/ass.v8n5p93.

Nadesan, M. H., & Sotirin, P. (1998). The romance and science of "breast is best": Discursive contradictions and contexts of breast-feeding choices. *Text and Performance Quarterly, 18,* 217–232.

Ochsner Clinic Department of Pediatrics. M is for the many joys I'll bring mother.

Pollock, D. (1999). *Telling bodies/performing birth: Everyday narratives of childbirth.* New York: Columbia University Press.

Robledo, D. (2012). Integrative use of social media in health communication. *Online Journal of Communication and Media Technologies, 2,* 77–95.

Rosin, H. (2009, April). The case against breast-feeding. *The Atlantic.* Retrieved February 11, 2013, from http://www.theatlantic.com/magazine/archive/2009/04/the-case-against-breast-feeding/307311.

Shoemaker, D. (2011). Mamafesto!: Why superheroes wear capes. *Text and Performance Quarterly, 32,* 190–202.

Smith, J. P., & Ellwood, M. (2011). Feeding patterns and emotional care in breastfed infants. *Social Indicators Research, 101,* 227–231. doi 10.1007/s11205-010-9657-9.

Taylor, E. N., & Wallace, L. E. (2012). Breastfeeding promotion and the problem of guilt. In P. H. Smith, B. L. Hausman, & M. Labbock (Eds.), *Beyond health, beyond choice: Breastfeeding constraints and realities* (pp. 193–202). New Brunswick, NJ: Rutgers University Press.

Weimer, D. R. (2005). Summary of state breastfeeding laws. In S. W. Ying (Ed.), *Breastfeeding: laws and societal impact* (pp. 57–77). New York: Nova Science.

Wilson, R. (2009). Is having more than 2 children an unspoken taboo? *Chronicle of Higher Education 55,* 41. B16–19.

Wolynn, T. (2012). Using social media to promote and support breastfeeding. *Breastfeeding Medicine, 7,* 364–365. doi: 10.1089/bfm.2012.0085.

7 Comparing Chinese Immigrant Women with Caucasian Women on Maternal Health Communication with Healthcare Providers

Findings from the Los Angeles Mommy and Baby (LAMB) Survey

Yuping Mao and Lu Shi

Introduction

In the United States, Chinese immigrants have been the fastest growing ethnic minority population over the past two decades and are the second largest immigrant group in the after Mexicans (Camarota, 2007). In 2010, the Chinese immigrant population in the United States reached 1.8 million (McCabe, 2012). Chinese immigrant women's health issues have become an increasingly important social issue as this population grows. In the U.S. society, the Chinese are perceived as "the model minority" with higher income and educational levels than the U.S. national average. However, in the U.S. context Chinese immigrant women's health communication might not be as effective as their Caucasian counterparts. For instance, researchers found that the loss of extended social networks and language barriers are the two primary reasons Chinese immigrants have difficulties in accessing health information (Ahmad et al., 2004). Yu, Huang, and Singh (2004) reported that many Chinese immigrant families do not benefit from needed services that may be available in their community owing to the lack of access to and understanding of the U.S. healthcare system. Thus, there is a need of research to understand Chinese immigrant women's experiences of communication for health information.

For a woman, pregnancy can be an exciting experience, but it is also a time when she requires more health consultation with healthcare providers. For both practitioners and researchers, it is important to hear the voices of and understand the health communication preferences of minority groups who have been traditionally marginalized from mainstream health communication discourse (Johnson et al., 2004). Understanding Chinese immigrant women's health communication during various maternal stages could provide rich information on their health needs and their health communication challenges.

Through analyzing the Los Angeles Mommy and Baby (LAMB) 2007 survey, this research attempts to explore the content of doctor–patient communication during women's pre-pregnancy, prenatal, and postnatal physician visits. We also discuss the similarities and differences between Chinese immigrant women and Caucasian women in their information exchange with their healthcare providers. The current U.S. medical system and medical education are based primarily on an understanding of the Caucasian "majority" population, and so might not fully reflect minority and immigrant population's health needs rooted in their cultural values. Findings from our study can provide useful information for practitioners who work on immigrant women's maternal health issues when they design health programs and initiatives to better serve those women's specific needs.

Literature Review

Individuals use different strategies to cope with health communication challenges, and different cultural groups have their health communication preferences. Health information seeking and avoiding are a balancing act for individuals who need to achieve multiple goals such as improving health outcome and reducing uncertainty (Brashers, Goldsmith, & Hsieh, 2002). Minority groups tend to adopt a passive pattern of information seeking (Chatman, 1996). Seeking health information that sometimes includes jargons rarely used in daily interactions can be challenging for Chinese immigrants. Chinese immigrant women in Canada identify linguistic difficulty, time pressure, and differences in the healthcare systems between China and Canada as important barriers to effective health information seeking (Ahmad et al., 2004). Therefore, they want health information in Chinese delivered through different means such as newspapers, television, and pamphlets. Among different media formats, Chinese immigrant women prefer receiving health information from printed materials. In addition, social networks have been found to be significant information sources for vulnerable populations (Liu, 1995; Metoyer-Duran, 1993). Informal social networks are especially helpful for immigrants experiencing language and cultural barriers (Hernandez-Plaza, Pozo, & Alonso-Morillejo, 2004), and immigration populations rely more on their informal social networks than formal institutions and organizations (Litwak, 1985).

Among different ways of seeking health information, the interaction between patients and healthcare providers remains important. Doctor–patient communication occurs in a particular sociocultural context that shapes health information-seeking behavior, interpreting, and understanding (Pachter, 1994). Cross-cultural communication issues between healthcare providers and receivers can further complicate health information seeking and avoiding (Goldsmith, 2001). When individuals from family-centered cultures (e.g., Chinese culture) interact with healthcare providers in the United States, information seeking or avoiding involves a complex coordination among healthcare providers, patients, patients' family, and, sometimes, interpreters (Brashers et al., 2002). Chinese cultural values and characteristics, such as Confucian, holism, collectivism, and emphasis on family relationship, all impact Chinese immigrants' health communication with their healthcare providers (Cheung et al., 2005). Furthermore, research has found that patients and healthcare providers may have different ideas about what kind of information is needed (Hines, Babrow, Badzek, & Moss, 2001). In the interactions between Chinese immigrants and their U.S. healthcare providers, the discrepancy between each other's understanding of information needs might be bigger than that in an interaction between an American patient and an American healthcare provider, owing to the cultural differences. This might influence the choice of health topics discussed during medical visits. There might be some important topics that Chinese immigrant women would rather not discuss with their healthcare providers; thus, those important voices might be unknown or underestimated by their healthcare providers.

Based on the above literature review, factors such as cultural differences and language barriers may lead to different information-seeking and avoiding behaviors between Chinese immigrant women and their Caucasian counterparts in their conversations with healthcare providers. It is logical to worry that mainstream services may not be compatible with the cultural needs and orientation of ethnic minority groups such as Chinese (Devore & Schlesinger, 1999). However, little is known about Chinese immigrant women's health communication with their U.S. healthcare providers. This study could contribute to the literature on minority women's health communication with their healthcare providers by comparing the topics discussed during maternal visits by Chinese immigrant women with those topics discussed by Caucasian women. In medical visits before, during, and after a pregnancy, health communication between women and their healthcare providers influences maternal and child health for many years to come. We hope our report on findings from analysts such as Gilligan and Furness (2006) and Yu (2006) will help practitioners develop culturally sensitive services to immigrant women, providing better maternal and family health outcomes.

Method

The LAMB survey is a population-based survey with multilevel clustered sampling. The survey was developed by the Maternal, Child, and Adolescent Health Programs of Los Angeles County. The purpose of the survey was to examine maternal and child health indicators such as prenatal care, health behavior during pregnancy, and postnatal recovery. The 2007 LAMB survey was conducted among new mothers who had a live birth in the Los Angeles County 4 to 7 months before. To reach respondents from different cultures, the surveys were conducted in different languages including English,

Spanish, and Chinese. Tailored cover letters, incentives, multiple mailings, and nonrespondent follow-up were used to increase the response rate. In total, 4518 of the 12,675 women reached by the multilevel sampling completed the survey, which resulted in a response rate of 35.6%. In our analysis, we focused on the survey results from Chinese immigrant women and Caucasian women. For the purpose of this study, we only analyzed survey items related to women's communication with their healthcare providers during their prepregnancy visit, prenatal checkup, and postnatal checkup.

Sample

In our sample, the Chinese immigrant women had lived in the United States an average of about 15 years. The average family income of Chinese immigrant women participants was slightly higher than that of the Caucasian women participants, which reflects national demographic characteristics. Participants only filled out the sections of the survey that were relevant to their experience, so some participants could skip questions on doctor's visits at the prepregnancy stage or other stages if they did not make the visits. Therefore, the samples are different in the analysis of women's health communication with their healthcare providers at different stages; see Table 7.1. Overall, Chinese immigrant women participants in this study were slightly older and had a higher educational background than the average.

Table 7.1 Sample Information

Key information	Prepregnancy	Prenatal	Postnatal
Number of Chinese immigrant women	59	151	142
Number of Caucasian women	193	535	490
Total number of participants	252	686	632
Average age of Chinese immigrant women	33.6	32.9	33.0
Average age of Caucasian women	31.8	30.1	30.4
Percentage of Chinese immigrant women with a Bachelor's degree or higher	74.6%	70.2%	70.4
Percentage of Caucasian women with a Bachelor's degree or higher	58.0%	41.9%	44.3%

Measurement

The 2007 LAMB survey documented the respondent's discussion with health professionals by asking her whether a doctor or a nurse had talked to her about certain health topics during the prepregnancy visit, her prenatal care checkup, and postnatal checkup. The questions that we analyzed were all categorical. Participants were asked to check whether their healthcare providers talked to them about certain health issues during their visits at different stages.

The question about prepregnancy visits was: "Think about the times you saw a doctor or nurse in the six months before you got pregnant. Did your provider talk to you about these topics to get you ready for pregnancy?" The respondents could check "Yes" or "No" on the following topics: multivitamin or folic acid supplements, healthy weight for pregnancy, immunizations, nutrition, smoking, blood sugar, blood pressure, existing medical conditions (e.g., asthma, anemia), gums and teeth, domestic violence, anxiety or depression, birth control, genetic screening, and lead and/or mercury exposure.

The question about the prenatal checkup was: "During the checkup, did your doctor or nurse talk to you about any of the following? Check all that apply." The respondents could check "Yes" or "No" on the following topics: birth control, breastfeeding, baby's sleeping position, loss of weight gained during pregnancy, blood sugar, blood pressure, domestic violence/child abuse, anxiety, depression, smoking, drinking alcohol, drug use, and childhood lead exposure.

The question about postnatal checkup was: "During the checkup, did your doctor or nurse talk to you about any of the following: Check all that apply." The respondents could check "Yes" or "No" on the following topics: birth control, breastfeeding, baby's sleeping position, loss of weight gained during pregnancy, blood sugar and blood pressure, domestic violence/child abuse, anxiety, depression, smoking, drinking alcohol, drug use, and childhood lead exposure.

Data Analysis

Using SAS 9.2's PROC FREQ statement, we compared the key checkup discussion content between Chinese and Caucasian respondents. Chi-square tests were performed to check the statistical significance of the differences.

Results

Part of the results about prepregnancy visits confirmed the general perception of Chinese as "the model minority," since Chinese immigrant women were significantly more likely to discuss physical health issues such as immunizations (57.1% vs. 37.2%, $p < .05$), stopping smoking (53.7% vs. 35.4%, $p < .05$), and blood sugar (52.4% vs. 35.7%, $p < .05$) than Caucasian women (see Table 7.2). No medical or physical health topic was found to be discussed significantly less by Chinese immigrant women with their healthcare providers than by Caucasian women. However, Chinese immigrant women were significantly less likely to discuss more socially and culturally related topics such as birth control (42.9% vs. 61.3%, $p < .05$) and domestic violence (5.1% vs. 17.6%, $p < .05$) with their healthcare providers than Caucasian women (see Table 7.2).

Table 7.2 Discussion of Health Topics among Chinese and Caucasian Women during Prepregnancy Visits

Race of mother	Multivitamin/ Folic acid		Healthy weight for pregnancy		Immunizations		Nutrition		Stop smoking		Blood sugar		Blood pressure	
	No	Yes	No	Yes	No	Yes	No	Yes	No	Yes	No	Yes	No	Yes
Caucasian percentage (%)	9.0	91.0	38.7	61.3	62.8	37.2	30.0	70.0	64.6	35.4	64.3	35.7	64.5	35.5
Chinese percentage (%)	8.8	91.2	29.2	70.8	42.9	57.1	16.7	83.3	46.3	53.7	47.7	52.4	52.5	47.5
Total percentage (%)	8.9	91.1	36.6	63.4	58.6	41.4	27.1	72.9	60.6	39.4	60.8	39.2	62.1	38.0
Chi-square statistic	F	P	F	P	F	$P*$	F	P	F	$P*$	F	$P*$	F	P
	0.002	0.96	1.46	0.23	5.43	0.02	3.37	0.07	4.49	0.03	3.88	0.04	1.95	0.16

Race of mother	Birth control		Medical conditions		Gums and teeth		Domestic violence		Anxiety/ Depression		Genetic screening		Lead and/or mercury	
	No	Yes	No	Yes	No	Yes	No	Yes	No	Yes	No	Yes	No	Yes
Caucasian percentage (%)	38.8	61.3	64.9	35.1	68.0	32.0	82.4	17.6	71.2	28.8	50.6	49.4	75.0	25.0
Chinese percentage (%)	57.1	42.9	69.2	30.8	57.1	42.9	94.9	5.1	85.4	14.6	37.8	62.2	67.5	32.5
Total percentage (%)	42.6	57.4	65.8	34.2	65.6	34.4	85.0	15.0	74.2	25.8	47.7	52.3	73.4	26.6
Chi-square statistic	F	$P*$	F	P	F	P	F	$P*$	F	P	F	P	F	P
	4.60	0.03	0.26	0.61	1.71	0.19	3.75	0.05	3.37	0.07	2.31	0.13	0.91	0.34

*$P < 0.05$; **$P < 0.01$; ***$P < 0.001$

During prenatal care visits, Chinese immigrant women were significantly less likely than Caucasian women to have talked with doctors or nurses about birth control (55.9% vs. 71.5%, $p < .05$), flu vaccination (32.6% vs. 48.5%, $p < .05$), and what to do if labor started early (66.4% vs. 86.0%) (see Table 7.3). This same racial difference in discussions about birth control (74.8% vs. 92.3%, $p < .001$) remained during these women's postnatal checkup (see Table 7.4), when Chinese mothers were also significantly less likely than Caucasian mothers to have discussed with doctors or nurses about their baby's sleeping position (33.7% vs. 46.5%, $p < .05$), breastfeeding (68% vs. 81.3%, $p < .001$) and maternal weight loss (33.0% vs. 43.8%, $p < .05$) (see Table 7.4).

Tables 7.5 and 7.6 document the racial differences in discussing domestic abuse, substance abuse, and mental health. Chinese immigrant women were significantly less likely than Caucasian women to have talked about domestic abuse (15.2% vs. 26.0%, $p < .01$) and stopping drug use (41.1% vs. 50.6%, $p < .05$) during their prenatal care visits (Table 7.5). Chinese immigrant women were also significantly less likely to have discussed anxiety (11.5% vs. 24.7%, $p < .05$) and depression (15.6% vs. 42.2%, $p < .05$) than Caucasian women during their postnatal checkups (Table 7.6). Besides the above statistically significant findings, it is also worth noting the general pattern that Chinese immigrant women were less likely than Caucasian women to discuss mental health, family violence, and substance abuse issues that are highly related to social norm and culture. During prenatal visits, Chinese immigrant women were reported to be less likely to have discussed issues such as anxiety/depression, HIV testing, stopping smoking, drinking, and drug use with their healthcare providers than Caucasian women. During postnatal visits, Chinese immigrant women reportedly were less likely to have discussed domestic/child abuse, stopping smoking, drinking, and drug use with their healthcare providers than Caucasian women.

Discussion

Maternity can be stressful for both women and their families. Although Chinese culture is a collectivist culture and American healthcare providers might assume that Chinese people tend to have a strong association with their communities, overseas Chinese are far away and disconnected from their social networks in China. Compared with Caucasian American women, Chinese immigrant women in the United States may have greater need of social and psychological support during their pregnancies.

The survey reveals that an important communication gap between Chinese immigrant women and their healthcare providers during their prenatal and postnatal stages lies in their lack of communicative effort to seek social and psychological help from healthcare providers. Our survey showed that Chinese immigrant women were less likely to discuss some psychological

Table 7.3 Discussion of Physical Health Topics among Chinese and Caucasian Women during Prenatal Visits

Race of mother	Birth control		Breastfeeding		Seat Belt		Weight gain		Flu vaccine		Early labor		Lead exposure	
	No	Yes	No	Yes	No	Yes	No	Yes	No	Yes	No	Yes	No	Yes
Caucasian Percentage (%)	28.5	71.5	30.7	69.3	63.3	36.7	18.8	81.2	51.5	48.5	14.0	86.0	74.4	25.6
Chinese Percentage (%)	44.1	55.9	35.4	64.6	71.7	28.3	19.7	80.3	67.4	32.6	33.6	66.4	78.4	21.6
Total Percentage (%)	31.8	68.2	31.7	68.3	65.2	34.8	19.0	81.0	54.9	45.1	18.2	81.8	75.2	24.8
Chi-square statistics	F	P***	F	P	F	P	F	P	F	P**	F	P***	F	P
	12.6	0.0004	1.15	0.28	3.5	0.06	0.06	0.81	10.8	0.001	28.9	<.0001	0.89	0.35

*$P < 0.05$; **$P < 0.01$; ***$P < 0.001$

Table 7.4 Discussion of Physical Health Topics among Chinese and Caucasian Women during Postnatal Visits

Race of mother	Birth control		Breastfeeding		Baby sleep position		Losing weight		Blood sugar		Blood pressure		Lead exposure	
	No	Yes	No	Yes	No	Yes	No	Yes	No	Yes	No	Yes	No	Yes
Caucasian percentage (%)	7.7	92.3	18.8	81.3	53.5	46.5	56.2	43.8	77.0	23.0	77.7	22.3	85.0	15.0
Chinese percentage (%)	25.2	74.8	32.0	68.0	66.3	33.7	67.0	33.0	82.5	17.5	84.7	15.3	91.7	8.3
Total percentage (%)	11.8	88.2	21.9	78.1	56.4	43.6	58.7	41.3	78.2	21.8	79.3	20.7	86.5	13.5
Chi-square statistics	F	P***	F	P***	F	P*	F	P*	F	P	F	P	F	P
	23.38	<.001	8.15	<0.001	5.10	0.02	3.73	0.05	1.33	0.25	2.22	0.14	2.85	0.09

*$P < 0.05$; **$P < 0.01$; ***$P < 0.001$

Table 7.5 Discussion of Mental Health, Family Violence and Substance Abuse among Chinese and Caucasian Women during Prenatal Visits

Race of mother	Domestic abuse		Anxiety/ Depression		HIV testing		Stopping smoking		Stopping drinking		Stopping drug use	
	No	Yes	No	Yes	No	Yes	No	Yes	No	Yes	No	Yes
Caucasian percentage (%)	74.0	26.0	48.4	51.6	33.7	66.3	51.5	48.5	48.9	51.1	49.4	50.6
Chinese percentage (%)	84.8	15.2	56.7	43.3	39.1	60.9	51.0	49.0	52.9	47.1	58.9	41.1
Total percentage (%)	76.3	23.7	50.2	49.8	34.8	65.2	51.4	48.6	49.8	50.2	51.4	48.6
Chi-square statistics	F	P**	F	P	F	P	F	P	F	P	F	P*
	7.02	0.008	3.04	0.08	1.43	0.23	.008	0.92	0.68	0.41	6.9	0.03

$* P < 0.05$; $** P < 0.01$; $*** P < 0.001$

Table 7.6 Discussion of Mental Health, Family Violence and Substance Abuse among Chinese and Caucasian Women during Postnatal Visits

Race of mother	Domestic/child abuse		Anxiety		Depression		Stopping smoking		Stopping drinking		Stopping drug use	
	No	Yes	No	Yes	No	Yes	No	Yes	No	Yes	No	Yes
Caucasian percentage (%)	88.3	11.7	75.3	24.7	57.8	42.2	92.3	7.7	92.6	7.4	93.8	6.2
Chinese percentage (%)	94.8	5.2	88.5	11.5	84.4	15.6	95.8	4.2	95.8	4.2	95.8	4.2
Total percentage (%)	89.8	10.2	78.3	21.7	63.8	36.2	93.1	6.9	93.3	6.7	94.2	5.8
Chi-square statistic	F	P	F	P**	F	P***	F	P	F	P	F	P
	3.49	0.06	7.64	0.01	22.80	<.0001	1.47	0.23	1.26	0.26	0.58	0.45

$* P < 0.05$; $** P < 0.01$; $*** P < 0.001$

issues such as postnatal depression, and family issues such as birth control with healthcare providers than Caucasian women. Chinese immigrant women were significantly less likely to discuss birth control during pre-pregnancy, prenatal, and postnatal visits with their doctors, which could be explained by the Chinese collective culture mandating that "most problems among family members are handled within the family and controlled by the extended family, because social and legal structures recognize the family as a unit, but not individuals" (Zhan, 2002). It is possible that Chinese immigrant women are reluctant to discuss with their healthcare providers issues that are considered sensitive or private in Chinese culture, but it is also possible that healthcare providers tend not to bring up those topics in their discussion with Chinese immigrant women based on their preexisting understanding of Chinese culture. However, it is very clear that mental health, psychological, and family violence issues are important for women's health. Both healthcare providers and Chinese immigrant women should be trained and reminded to confront those issues instead of avoiding them in medical visits. Meanwhile, it is important for healthcare providers to make an effort to build trust in their relationship with Chinese immigrant women, which could be a decisive factor in Chinese immigrant women's choice to discuss those culturally and socially sensitive issues with their healthcare providers.

Furthermore, our findings show that Chinese immigrant women were significantly less likely than Caucasian women to discuss postnatal depression, a widely existing mental problem at the postnatal stage, with their healthcare providers. It is reasonable to doubt whether the current U.S. American health system has sufficiently met the mental health needs of Chinese immigrant women. Practitioners could consider adopting suggestions on meeting the Chinese community's mental health needs in other Western countries. Li, Logan, Yee, and Ng (1999) provided the following suggestions to improve satisfying the Chinese community's mental health needs in England: (1) Maximize the effectiveness of health professional–patient contacts through training for health service staff and access to health advocates; (2) promote a better understanding of mental illness within the Chinese community; (3) ensure that the health system include health professionals with bilingual skillsand use those professionals to the best effect.

Practitioners should also consider some other media initiatives to supplement the interpersonal communication gap between Chinese immigrant women and their healthcare oroviders. An online discussion board has been used by overseas Chinese immigrant women for maternal health issues. A content analysis of online discussion boards on maternal issues shows that the following topics are popular among overseas Chinese immigrant women: pregnancy and delivery, medical issues, maternal and baby product, doctors and hospitals, family relationship, and active attempts to conceive (Mao, Qian, & Starosta, 2010). Online platforms that allow more anonymous disclosure could be used to facilitate open discussion on culturally and socially sensitive topics among Chinese immigrant women. Overall, to provide maternal health support for Chinese immigrant women, practitioners should consider using various channels such as "face-to-face encounters (e.g., personal conversations, support groups, and healthcare interactions) and mediated communication (e.g., television, internet websites, email, pamphlets, self-help books, and health magazines)," as suggested by Brashers et al. (2002).

Language may not be a major obstacle for doctor–patient communication on medical and physical health topics, but all the same it might constrain communication on mental and psychological health. Our findings showed only minor differences between Chinese immigrant women and Caucasian women on physical health and medical topics discussed in their maternal visits with healthcare practitioners. Although conversations on medical issues may involve some jargon that people do not use in their daily life, Chinese immigrant women might have tried to learn those words before they went to see their doctors or nurses. However, language barriers might contribute to the overall pattern showing that Chinese immigrant women were less likely to discuss mental health, psychological, and family health issues with healthcare providers. The limited English-language proficiency could constrain Chinese immigrant women's ability to freely discuss complex and sensitive issues that are more closely associated with cultural and social value. Therefore, practitioners could consider providing mental, psychological, and family health service in Chinese and adopting a community-based approach. Collaboration with nonprofit agencies among the Chinese immigrant community could help overcome challenges associated with language and cultural differences.

Conclusion

Through an analysis of the 2007 LAMB survey, this research study showed both similarities and differences in topics being discussed in Chinese immigrant women's and Caucasian women's maternal visits with their healthcare providers in the United States. There were few and only minor differences between Chinese immigrant women and Caucasian women on those physical health topics and medical topics that they discussed with their healthcare providers, but major differences existed in topics involving mental, psychological, and family health. Overall, Chinese immigrant women were less likely to discuss mental, psychological, and family health issues with healthcare providers than their Caucasian counterparts. This study suggests that the current healthcare system in the United States should be aware of the group differences between Chinese immigrant women and Caucasian women and design culturally sensitive programs to provide social and psychological help to Chinese immigrant women during their prenatal and postnatal stages.

References

Ahmad, F., Shik, A., Vanza, R., Cheung, A., George, U., & Stewart, D.E. (2004). Popular health promotion strategies among Chinese and East Indian immigrant women. *Women and Health, 40*(1), 21–40. DOI: 10.1300/J013v40n01_02.

Brashers, D. E., Goldsmith D. J., & Hsieh, E. (2002). Information seeking and avoiding in health contexts. *Human Communication Research, 28*(2), 258–271. DOI: 10.1093/hcr/28.2.258.

Camarota, S. (2007). Immigrants in the United States, 2007: A profile of America's foreign-born population. *The Center for Immigration Studies.* Retrieved September 15, 2015, from http://www.cis.org/immigrants_profile_2007.

Chatman, E. A. (1996). The impoverished life-world of outsiders. *Journal of the American Society for Information Science, 47*(2), 193–206. DOI: 10.1002/(SICI)1097-4571(199603)47:3<193::AID-ASI3>3.0.CO;2-T.

Cheung, R., Nelson, W., Advincula, L., Cureton, V. Y., & Canham, D. L. (2005). Understanding the culture of Chinese children and families. *Journal of School Nursing, 21*(3), 3–9. DOI: 10.1177/10598405050210010301.

Devore, W., & Schlesinger, E. G. (1999). *Ethnic-sensitive social work practice.* Boston: Allyn and Bacon.

Gilligan, P., & Furness, S. (2006). The role of religion and spirituality in social work practice: Views and experiences of social workers and students. *British Journal of Social Work, 36*(4), 617–637. DOI: 10.1093/bjsw/bch252.

Goldsmith, D. J. (2001). A normative approach to the study of uncertainty and communication. *Journal of Communication, 51,* 514–533. DOI: 10.1111/j.1460-2466.2001.tb02894.x.

Hernandez-Plaza, S., Pozo, C., & Alonso-Morillejo, E. (2004). The role of informal social support in needs assessment: Proposal and application of a model to assess immigrants' needs in the South of Spain. *Journal of Community and Applied Social Psychology, 14,* 284–298. DOI: 10.1002/casp.782.

Hines, S. C., Babrow, A. S., Badzek, L., & Moss, A. H. (2001). From coping with life to coping with death: Problematic integration for the seriously ill elderly. *Health Communication,13,* 327–342. DOI: 10.1207/S15327027HC1303_6.

Johnson, J. L., Bootorff, J. L., Browne, A. J., Grewal, S., Hilton, B. A., & Clarke, H. (2004). Othering and being othered in the context of health care services. *Health Communication, 16,* 253–272. DOI: 10.1207/S15327027HC1602_7.

Li, P-L, Logan, S., Yee, L., & Ng, S. (1999). Barriers to meeting the mental health needs of the Chinese community. *Journal of Public Health Medicine, 21*(1), 74–80. DOI: 10.1093/pubmed/21.1.74.

Litwak, E. (1985). *Helping the elderly: The complementary roles of informal networks and formal systems.* New York: Guilford Press.

Liu, M. (1995). Ethnicity and information seeking. *Reference Library, 49*(50), 123–134. DOI: 10.1300/J120v23n49_09.

Mao, Y., Qian, Y., & Starosta, W. (2010). A cross-cultural comparison of American and overseas Chinese prenatal and postnatal women's online social support behavior in two online message boards. In J-R. Park & E. Abels (Eds.), *Interpersonal relations and social patterns in communication technologies: Discourse norms, language structures and cultural variables* (pp. 331–353). Hershey, PA: IGI Global.

McCabe, K. (2012). Chinese immigrants in the United States. Retrieved September 15, 2015, from: http://migrationpolicy.org/article/chinese-immigrants-united-states.

Metoyer-Duran, C. (1993). The information and referral process in culturally diverse communities. *Reference Quarter (RQ), 32*(3), 359–371. DOI: www.jstor.org/stable/25829307.

Pachter, L. M. (1994). Culture and clinical care: Folk illness beliefs and behaviors and their implications for health care delivery. *Journal of the American Medical Association, 271,* 690–694. DOI: 10.1001/jama.1994.03510330068036.

Yu, S. M., Huang, Z. J., & Singh, G. K. (2004). Health status and health services utilization among US Chinese, Asian Indian, Filipino, and other Asian/Pacific Islander children. *Pediatrics, 113,* 101–107. DOI: 10.1542/peds.113.1.101l.

Yu, W. K. (2006). Adaptation and tradition in the pursuit of good health: Chinese people in the UK—The implications for ethnic sensitive social work practice. *International Social Work, 49*(6), 757–766. DOI: 10.1177/0020872806070973.

Zhan, H. (2002). Chinese family and the state: Gender-role socialization and social control. *Sexual Health Exchange, 2002*(4), 7–10. DOI: 10.1111/j.1467-6443.1996.tb00187.x.

8 Japanese Women's Suicide and Depression under the Panopticon

Kimiko Akita

Introduction

All females in Japan suffer under *ie* (pronounced "*ee-eh*" and meaning *family* or *household*), a patriarchal family system rooted in Confucianism. The system requires that women subjugate themselves to fathers, husbands, and sons and persevere for the sake of their family. Women are expected to administer household affairs and raise and care for the children and the elderly, and resolve all emotional or relational issues for family. Under the *ie* system, a wife is expected to treat her husband's and his immediate family members' healthcare as more important than that of her own, of her parents, or of her maiden family. The domestic obligations delineated by *ie* may well lead the woman into *utsu* [depression]. *Ie*'s victims tend to suffer in silence, following the Confucian value of perseverance rather than reveal their *utsu*. They would not want to worry their family or to appear as a failure.

Utsu has been recognized in Japan as melancholia, the physical and mental condition of stagnation in vital energy, since at least the 16th century (Kitanaka, 2012) but has been considered a mental illness since the late 19th century, when Japanese psychiatrists replaced traditional medical ideas with German neuropsychiatry (p. 21). Perceived as mentally ill, a person with *utsu* is severely stigmatized and often misunderstood and mistreated, left without social and governmental support.

A danger of the *ie* system is that because a woman must represent for her husband's family, her social identity is not self-identity but the collective family-unit identity. Women identify themselves by the paternal (father's, husband's, or son's) *ie* (see Gordon, 2011, p. 371), which discourages her from seeking outside help. If a mother/wife is stigmatized, not only she and her maiden family, but also her husband, and his side of the family, as well as their children, will thus become socially stigmatized. An *utsu* patient's relatives also are likely to remain silent and/or stay away from the *utsu* patient to avoid possible stigmatization. An *utsu* mother/wife tries her best not to discredit her *ie* (family). A woman afflicted with *utsu* is likely to try to suppress her condition, and as a result, it often becomes too late for her or her family members to find out about a mother/wife's *utsu*.

For instance, Princess Masako, wife of the heir to Japan's imperial throne—but also a Harvard graduate and former diplomat—exemplifies a mother/wife of the highest *ie* class who has suffered in silence from *utsu*. Upon making it public in 2003, she gave up her official duties (Parry, 2008) 10 years after her marriage to Crown Prince Naruhito. *Newsweek* magazine had long since noted Masako's being stifled and silenced inside the palace (Bartholet, 1996). Under tremendous pressure from both the Imperial House and the public to conceive a boy, Masako underwent fertility treatment and a miscarriage but had a daughter, Princess Aiko, in 2001 (Takayama, 2001). The media have depicted Masako as lazy, selfish, and useless (Ryall, 2008). Kanji Nishio, a right-wing academic political commentator, blamed her maiden family for damaging the image of the Royal Family and suggested that the Prince divorce Masako (Parry, 2008). Masako's *utsu* remains serious, and she hardly appears in public (Ryall, 2012). And with the lack of understanding and support for an *utsu* mother/wife in Japan, it will take a long time for Masako to get well.

In this chapter, I first discuss how *ie* functions similar to Jeremy Bentham's 1787 "Panopticon" design (see Foucault, 1977), in which the behavior and linguistic style of Japanese women are under a constant and "unequal gaze" designed to control them. Then, in a case study of *ie* and *utsu*, I will give voice to two women I know very well: both victims of *utsu* and suicide attempts after years of striving to become an ideal *ie* mother/wife. One of them was my aunt, who developed *utsu* and hanged herself in 1998. The other is my mother, my aunt's younger sister, who cried profusely at my aunt's funeral, telling her dead spirit how stupid she was to kill herself and how precious life was. No one would have guessed, though, that my mother, who had always appeared to us as healthy, cheerful, and strong, would herself develop *utsu* and attempt suicide in 2009.

A Brief History of *Ie* in Early Modern and Modern Japan

Ie implies a patrimonial, patrilineal, patrilocal, patriarchal Japanese family system (Koyama, 1961; Kano, 1983; Mihalopoulos, 2009), as well as other social and business systems (Inoue, 2000; Kondo, 1990; Koyama, 1961; Plath, 1964). Primogenitary (i.e., oldest son as sole heir) patriarchy was a primary *ie* imperative. *Ie* confined women's spaces to the house while privileging men's roles both outside and inside the house. In the *ie* system, not only Confucian values of obedience and endurance, but also Confucian etiquette and deportment were required of women (Robertson, 1991). A woman with refined *ie* manners, deportment, speech, and material wealth (e.g., wearing beautiful *kimonos*) earned respect and status and helped maintain her family's reputation (Akita, 2009). *Ie* also encouraged women to compete with other women. Even today, the Japanese respect a woman of refined deportment and speech more than they do a woman of intelligence (Akita, 2005).

Social-class hierarchy as a crucial part of *ie* dates to the 17th century. The Tokugawa Shogunate controlled Japan during the Edo era (1603–1868), so continuation of the *shogun*'s *ie* meant continuity for the nation. The Edo government legitimized and enforced *ie* (Inoue, 2000; Koyama, 1961). The government designated a hierarchy of four social classes: *samurai* (warriors), the highest class; *hyakusho* (farmers), the second class; *shokunin* (artisans), the third class; and *shonin* (merchants), the lowest class (Hane, 1982; Kitche, 1995). The government defined farmers as second rank merely to appease them, but the majority of Japanese belonged to the farmer class, and most were peasants. The *ie* concept was first adopted and practiced by *samurai*, then trickled down to those who emulated the upper class; the landowner farmer (top farmer class) and merchant classes adopted *ie* (Akita, 2005, 2009). *Ie* promoted an illusionary image, which one tried to keep up with for the sake of one's *ie* status (Inoue, 2006; Kano, 1983). One was encouraged to become an *alterity*, an idealization of a person one was not (Inoue, 2006). Whereas the warrior class, the landowner farmer class, and the merchant class rigidly practiced *ie*, the lower classes (artisans and peasants) did not have to follow *ie*—and could not afford to anyway.

Upon the Meiji Restoration in 1868, the government eliminated social-class distinctions and legalized *ie* to replace the class system with a new hierarchy. Suddenly, all were social equals; however, an *ie* class competition arose immediately (Inoue, 2006; Kano, 1983) in which families sought to outdo others in education, occupation, and wealth. The gender hierarchy—men superior to women—also became more distinct. The Meiji state popularized the slogan "*ryosai kenbo*" ["Good Wife, Wise Mother"] to influence women to believe that their gender roles constituted civil service (Nolte & Hastings, 1991). A man inherited family property; a woman received only a dowry, which went to her husband and his family. A woman was taught to submit to men (husbands, fathers, sons), to endure, and to sacrifice her self. One endeavored to project a good *ie* image according to this new social status system. The higher one's former class, the more rigidly and perfectly one tried to perform one's expected social and domestic roles without tarnishing her or his *ie* image (Akita, 2005).

Until the end of World War II, *ie* legally controlled women, but *ie* as law was abolished in 1948 by the postwar constitution (Kano, 1983, p. 6). Its ideology, however, has remained dominant, and competition for status continues. In postwar Japan, the formerly lower classes who could not afford and did not practice the rigid *samurai* class rituals entered the race driven by consumerism (Goldstein-Gidoni, 1999). An individual's ancestral social class was no longer easily discernible, so formerly lower-class people could construct and maintain the façade of the higher *ie* class. A woman from a lower social class could achieve high social status by acting how what she thought an *okusama* (upper-class mother/wife) would behave, through demeanor, speech, and material wealth (Akita, 2005, 2009).

More pressure was placed on the formerly upper-class mother/wife who needed to outshine newcomers to the higher classes. Naturally, a very high *ie* mother/wife, such as Princess Masako, would have to watch her own behavior more carefully, as she would be subjected to more gazes and be scrutinized by the public even more. Kondo (1990) noted that "discourses on *ie* create definitions of proper human conduct and mature personhood, providing the pathways to fulfilling these life trajectories and offering specific kinds of punishments for transgressions" (p. 141).

The image of "good wife/wise mother" was diffused through TV and radio commercials and programs from the 1950s on. Manufacturers and retailers, abetted by the mass media's burgeoning advertising industry, seized this opportunity to idealize a mother or bride by promoting domestic products a mother/wife could use for her family: a TV, a washing machine, a refrigerator (see Akita, 2009). Because the stay-at-home mother was promoted as the *ie* ideal during the wars of the early and mid-20th century, the mother image became sanctified (Kano, 1989). Peace activists in the postwar years used the mother, not the single woman, as the ultimate peace symbol. As a result, women had to become mothers to be able to speak their minds politically in public and to gain public respect (p. 109). A mother/wife was respected because she took care of her family (husband, children, in-laws) and her husband's community, into which she had married. Since the economic growth in Japan in the 1970s, along with an increase in the number of stay-at-home mothers, the status of *ie* mother/wife (stay-at-home mother) has risen (Kano, 2007). Among women, living the *okusama* life, which was promoted by media, has become the ideal (Kano, 1983, p. 118).

Utsu in Japan

The number of patients being treated for *utsu* in Japan increased from 433,000 in 1996 to surpass 1 million in 2011 (Ministry of Health, Labour and Welfare, 2011), not including unreported *utsu* patients. *Utsu* is 60% more common among females than males (Ministry of Health, Labour and Welfare, 2010). The number of suicides among the Japanese—many suffering from *utsu*—passed 30,000 in 1998 and has remained steady since then (Ministry of Health, Labour and Welfare, 2010), three times the number of auto fatalities (Hirai, 2004). Japan's suicide rate was highest in a study of seven developed nations (Ministry of Health, Labour and Welfare, 2010).

Utsu came under greater attention in the 1990s (Kitanaka, 2012). Although the Ministry of Health, Labour, and Welfare began providing long-term care insurance for Japanese senior citizens in 2000, the government does not include *utsu* in this insurance coverage. A senior incapacitated by *utsu* receives no long-term state support. Without it, an *utsu* patient would be reluctant to seek, and unable to afford, treatment. Almost all psychiatric inpatient care units that treat *utsu* in Japan require the husband's (or another family member's) consent for a woman who wants to be treated. Unable to have her *utsu* treated discreetly, she is likely to be discouraged to seek help.

Those most susceptible to *utsu* are meticulous (anal retentive), responsible, serious, diligent, trustworthy, obedient, and of high morals standards (Ono, 2000, p. 37). Dr. Kozo Shimoda, a Japanese psychiatrist, states that meticulous, diligent, and responsible personalities could also trigger bipolar disorder (Ono, 2000, p. 37). Japanese women who aspire to the role of the perfect *ie* mother/wife are susceptible to *utsu* because *ie* prescriptions are exactly what might trigger *utsu*.

Although *utsu* is perceived and treated as an individual's mental problem in Japan, a patient with *utsu* may also lose some physical capabilities (Ono, 2000; Shimozono, 2004). Some *utsu* patients may lose sensitivity or control in their hands and legs, may become blind, or may lose all concentration (Shimozono, 2004, p. 3). *Utsu* patients' experiences are similar to the trauma suffered by combatants. After subsisting in a constantly fearful, stressful, and exhaustive environment, *utsu* patients break down mentally, emotionally, and physically, becoming virtually unrecognizable (p. 3). Symptoms of *utsu* are apathy; sudden change in eating habits; exhaustion, constant fatigue, and sleepiness; self-criticism and self-blame; inability to think, to decide, and to function; desire to die; and suicidal thoughts (Shimozono, 2004, p. 8).

Utsu and *Alterity*

Giving up her voice and her self, the typical dedicated *ie* mother/wife transforms herself into a commodity or an Other, *alterity*, someone other than herself (Inoue, 2006, pp. 47–56), an idealization of the mother/wife she is not. Through imitating her ideal woman, she becomes an Other. Taussig (1993) described the *mimetics of alterity* as "the nature that culture uses to create second nature, the faculty to copy, imitate, make models, explore difference, yield into and become Other" (p. xiii). When a mother/wife attempts to emulate *alterity*, she commodifies herself; effaces herself, and mutes her personal needs and desires. Her mimetic faculty allows her to "become and behave like something else." The ability to mime, and to mime well, in other words, is the capacity to Other" (p. 19). A mother/wife must stifle her emotions and critical thinking and transform herself into someone she is not; an illusionary person.

For any human to suppress emotion and to become a commodity would seem unbearable. It would likely lead to cognitive dissonance, schizophrenia, or self-destruction. Further, aiming to become *alterity*, an imaginary woman, would leave one frustrated, depressed, hopeless. In addition, the *ie*'s imposition of collective identity traps women—once any slight transgression of *ie* behavior is detected, not only the mother/wife becomes stigmatized, but also her husband and children. The very thought of that would deter her from any transgression; she is a prisoner under constant gaze. On the other hand, ironically, a prisoner could be praised or rewarded when her *ie* performance is a success. This becomes an incentive for prisoners to stay in their prisons. This double mode, binary division (Foucault, 1977, p. 199) traps the prisoners.

The Panopticon of *Ie* for Women

Japanese women are responsible for the life cycles of others as well as their own (Plath, 1980, p. 127). A mother/wife is expected to care for her ill husband, children, and in-laws. It is expected that she will outlive her husband and care for him on his sickbed and his deathbed. She would be perceived as a failure if she became *utsu*; it would evidence her lack of the perseverance demanded by *ie*. Often, a dedicated *ie* mother/wife is unaware of *utsu*; or it may be found too late for effective treatment because of prolonged neglect. The worst scenario occurs when that woman chooses suicide to stop the emotional pain and suffering, the gaze, the criticism, the stigma.

In *Discipline and Punish,* Foucault (1977) discussed how Bentham's design of the *panopticon* for prisons worked in modern society and how discipline developed a new economy and politics for individuals. I argue that Japanese women live as prisoners constantly under what Foucault called an "unequal gaze" in the panopticon of *ie*. Under *ie*, the prisoners are unaware that they are being watched by guards; but the guards are, in reality, the prisoners themselves. To prescribe and continually enforce values required to maintain *ie*, each prisoner becomes a guard, critically monitoring herself or himself, as well as one another, for any sign of anti-*ie* behavior (see Akita, 2005). Both men and women are prisoners/guards in *ie*'s dungeon, but women are the more able corrective guards and prisoners. A woman prisoner from the highest *ie* class must be the model prisoner and watch her own behavior especially carefully. Other common prisoners, such as lower *ie* class prisoners, expect so much of this high *ie* woman that they would scrutinize her constantly and more critically. That same woman from a lower *ie* class is under less scrutiny. The guards (spectators) do not care as much about what she does. Prisoners are disciplined and punished through their own, as well as others', corrective "unequal gaze."

Because prisoners cannot see most other prisoners in the *ie* panopticon, they can only imagine how they might be watched and how they are supposed to behave. According to Foucault (1977), the "unequal gaze" causes internalization of disciplinary individuality and the docile body required of its inmates. The more aware a woman is of being watched, the less likely she will be to break rules. Therefore, a high *ie* woman will be less likely to break *ie* rules. A woman such as Princess Masako exemplifies the docile body; she had to secretly try harder to act as the very best of the high-class *ie* mother/wife in her cell. However, the high *ie* woman image itself is imaginary and unattainable. The more a woman tries to attain the ideal image through repression and endurance, the more she suffers secretly because she will never reach the level expected of her. The greater her cognitive dissonance, the more likely and profound her *utsu* and her suicidal ideation. I argue that women who believe that they are of high *ie*—or women who attempt to achieve high *ie*—are more susceptible to *utsu* and suicide.

Temptation to Suicide

Suicide, to many Japanese, means the cleansing of the soul, of the defiled life, before going on to the next, clean life. Family and religious factors have the most influence in an elderly woman's suicide in Japan (Chandler & Tsai, 1993). Buddhism's teaching of reincarnation may inadvertently encourage the *utsu* mother/wife to end this life and start fresh to carry out leftover duties for her family. Buddhists believe that the spirits of the deceased "live" among the surviving family and participate as guardians in their everyday lives. Buddhism is closely connected with ancestor veneration (Gordon, 2011). For a dedicated *ie* mother/wife, suicide signifies her apology to her husband's ancestors for not fulfilling her familial duties: "Suicide, properly done, will … clear his name and reinstate his memory. American condemnation of suicide makes self-destruction only a desperate submission to despair, but the Japanese respect for it allows it to be an honorable and purposeful act" (Benedict, 1946, p. 166). Suicide, though largely conceived as an act of mental illness in the West, demonstrates self-respect (p. 290) as well as self-dignity to many in Japan. A model mother/wife might see suicide, her self-sacrifice, as proof that she is accepting and self-inflicting the punishment she deserves for failing to perform *ie* mother/wife.

Bushido (1909) is the first published book on Japanese culture written by a Japanese man in English. Ritual suicide was only for the upper-class *ie*, such as *samurai* seeking honor, to prove innocence, or to express loyalty to his master, according to *bushido* [the soul of Japan] (Nitobe, 1909). *Bushido*, which was based on Shinto, Buddhism, Confucianism, and Mencius, taught *samurai* to live fully. Inadvertent choice of death was considered to be cowardly, sneaky, and dirty. "It [Suicide] was an institution, legal and ceremonial. … refinement of self-destruction, and none could perform it without the utmost coolness of temper and composure of demeanor" (p. 116).

My Aunt and My Mother

I write now about two high *ie* women I know very well. Both strove to be a high *ie* mother/wife/daughter, eventually succumbed to *utsu*, and attempted suicide. My aunt Akie ["autumn harvest fortune"] succeeded. Her sister Yukie ["snow branch"]—my mother—survived but suffers from severe *utsu* and bipolar disorder. Both women represent the docile bodies, the model prisoners (Foucault, 1977), in the *ie* panopticon. Neither had any idea at the time that they were prisoners. They were simply obedient to *ie*. Years ago, when they were healthy, they would always say, "I must be going because my husband must wonder where I am," "I couldn't possibly sit down since

I know my husband is working very hard somewhere now," or "I couldn't possibly decide. I must ask my husband for his opinion." It was as if their husbands were always scrutinizing them even when they were not around.

Akie and Yukie, 10 years apart in age, never lived in the same house at the same time. Akie, born in 1926, was the first daughter of a landowner farmer's family in central Japan. My maternal grandparents were happy that her brother Tatsuo had been born first, ensuring that he would succeed as male head of the family. Akie's mother's maiden family had been left with no children and was eager to adopt from their relatives to sustain the family succession, the *ie*. Akie's maternal grandfather's will demanded the adoption of the second child born to Akie's family regardless of the sex. As a result, when Akie turned 4 years old, her parents were forced to give her away to Akie's aunt (Akie's mother's elder sister) and her husband.

That aunt, Tane, never warmed to Akie because she was a girl. Tane also felt jealousy toward Akie and Akie's mother because of the new line of succession in Tane's family. In 1946, when Akie turned 20, her former uncle and now stepfather died. Two weeks later, Akie's stepmother, Tane, and her relatives arranged for Akie to marry a man she had never met because Akie and Tane could not maintain their farm without a man's help. It was considered shameful for a farm or business to be managed by women without a man in charge. Because Buddhism prohibits eating meat right after a death in the family, Akie's wedding reception included only simple vegetable dishes. Her childhood dream of one day having a nice wedding did not matter.

Until 1947, any family property or fortune would have been officially transferred to the male master of the family. So, immediately after Akie's wedding, her family fortune was conveyed to her husband. From then on, he handled the family's finances. Akie's stepmother insisted on keeping both herself and Akie subordinate to Akie's husband because of his value as the only man in the family, who would help with the heavy farm work and, most important, help produce offspring. Akie's husband represented hope in perpetuating *ie*.

Akie and her husband worked as landowner farmers and raised one son and two daughters. After the daughters married, the son, Koichi, as heir-to-be, married. His wife moved in with Akie and her husband. Their daughter-in-law, Teruyo, was from the city and had a college degree but no experience farming. Akie and her husband continued to work the farm without help from their son and daughter-in-law, who worked at jobs in the city. Akie maintained the house, the garden, the Buddhist altar, and the family graveyard without her daughter-in-law's help.

Teruyo was a modern, outspoken woman and openly criticized Akie. Though surprised, my aunt kept silent and endured and continued to be nice to Teruyo to maintain *ie* and harmony. But even Teruyo's children mistreated the grandparents. Akie's husband disregarded his wife's concerns. Once, Akie suggested that the two families live in separate houses, but her husband rejected the idea, saying such an arrangement would stigmatize the family. Finally, when Akie could no longer endure the isolation and neglect, she committed suicide. During a half hour of free time while my uncle went to a barber, Akie found her opportunity and hanged herself from a tree at the entrance to her gorgeous, 100-year-old, wood-frame home, surrounded by a Japanese garden. In Akie's belief system, she went on to a life after death, the only place where she could enjoy any freedom. She left a note in hurried scribble, which my uncle found under a *zabuton* ["seating cushion"] in the living room after her wake.

> My dear family, thank you very much for taking care of me for all these years. Because of my illness, I do not wish to burden you anymore. So, I am going away now. I am sorry that I have caused any trouble to you. Akie

Although my aunt's health was not perfect, she was healthy enough to work on the farm. People who had known about her difficult and unhappy life knew that my aunt lied—even in her last testament—to save face for her family members. Akie's family hid the fact of her suicide from their neighbors.

Akie's death was a terrible blow to me and to my mother, who had tried to comfort Akie over the years. We never understood her problem to be that serious. At least, we thought her husband was taking good care of her. It was only after her suicide that my mother and I realized that my aunt had repressed herself and never shared the problems in her marriage.

Until 2001, no one in Akie's neighborhood would speak about Akie or her death, and it took two years for me to get information about Akie, her marriage, and her suicide. Long the ethnographer at this point in my life, I obtained this information through a careful, unobtrusive investigation with the help of my mother, who was always Akie's very sociable younger sister and who knew Akie's neighbors and relatives. To give voice to my aunt, I first published her suicide in 2003 (see Akita, 2003). Researching my aunt's life was an awakening for me because I came to realize that I had been allowing myself to live under the same pervasive, invisible power of *ie* and to let *ie* dictate my life. My aunt's suicide energized me. Determined to speak for voiceless women like my aunt, I returned to the United States to study gender and generational issues more intensively than ever and to get my Ph.D. in 1998 (see Akita, 2006).

My Mother's Imprisoned Life

Both my paternal and maternal families are similar-sized landowner families, dating back more than 250 years. My family has lived on the same property since the mid-Edo era, in the 1700s. My mother, Yukie, received good bridal training. She told me:

> The landowners' daughters received bridal training, such as sewing lessons, the tea ceremony, and flower arranging, and they married by

arrangement. We had to bring a dowry and hold extravagant wedding ceremonies. But peasants' daughters could marry for love or elope without any bridal training. They did not need a dowry or even a wedding. My sisters and I used to envy them for their simple and easy life, their emancipation and mobility.

My parents' marriage was arranged, a practice emulating that of the upper-class people in those days. My mother was not impressed with my father at her initial meeting, but she felt obliged to accept the offer arranged by her aging parents. She did not care for my father, but her marrying would reduce her parents' financial burden. From the start, my paternal grandmother mistreated my mother. One reason was that my mother's maiden family owned larger properties, a sign of status. In addition, my mother was more educated than my father. When I was very young, my mother would talk about history and recite *haiku*. Displaying her intelligence always angered my father to violence, which would shut her up quickly.

My father did not want to take a salaried job, even when agricultural prices dropped in the early 1960s. He bought chickens but made my mother take care of them and sell eggs from our home. My father finally got a full-time job as a plumber, but his salary was not enough. My mother took charge of the farm, the chickens, and the eggs and took care of us children and our paternal grandmother. Times were hard for us. So my mother took a full-time job at a factory in 1974, in addition to managing and working the farm. My paternal grandmother said to my mother: "You've been fooling around at home. You'd better start working."

My mother's workload was enormous. She awakened before the chickens or anyone in my family. She worked in the vegetable or rice fields in the early morning, fed the chickens, then worked at the factory from 8 am to 7 pm. She would grab a bite of food and run to whatever was next. After dinner, my mother cleaned eggs and delivered them to hospitals and restaurants, working until 1 or 2 am. On weekends, she worked the fields all day until late in the night. I used to bike to the fields late at night and beg my mother to stop and come home and eat dinner. I turned angry and sad whenever I saw my mother, exhausted, fall asleep as she ate or while bathing in a tub. My father and my grandmother had gone to their rooms by 8 pm and were asleep long before my mother made it to bed. Meanwhile, my mother never told anyone, even her own mother, about my father's physical abuse.

She quit the factory job and started a real estate business in 1991, turning much of our vast farmlands, which my father had inherited, into rental apartments, parking lots, and warehouses. My paternal grandmother died at the age of 96 in 1986. Relieved of the burden of constantly caring for her, my mother finally agreed to obtain a passport and started to enjoy overseas trips with me. My father stopped working altogether and relied on the income from my mother's real estate business. My mother still took care of the house, the garden, our ancestors' graveyard, and my father. My two sisters, who left our family home when they got married, never helped. Since 1998, I have lived in the United States, far away from my mother.

By October 2008, Yukie fell ill from exhaustion brought on mostly by taking care of my father, whose physical violence escalated because of his Alzheimer's disease. I flew to Japan, stayed with Yukie, and taught her how to use Skype so that we could stay in daily contact across a great distance, which cheered her up. Yukie recovered during my visit. Then, in the summer of 2009, Yukie suddenly contacted me and begged me to move back to Japan; then she just as suddenly told me to stay in the United States. I was confused. As I prepared to move back to Japan anyway, I found out—purely by accident—that Yukie had attempted suicide on October 13, 2009. No one had told me about it at the time. I found out much later, when I visited my mother next month that she had cut herself deeply but survived.

Yukie left a will similar to what her sister Akie had written in 1998: full of self-criticism and self-blame and apologizing for her failure as a wife and mother. She plunged a kitchen knife into her stomach in front of the Buddhist altar where she had sat at least twice a day every day since she married into her husband's family. It was where Yukie had sat as a newly-wed in 1959 and placed her fingers together in utmost respect to my father's ancestors, introducing herself, pledging that she would try her best to be the ideal wife and mother, and asking for permission to be buried with them upon her death.

My father and my two sisters mistreated Yukie during the months of her recovery. They were upset for being stigmatized. Her suicide attempt exposed problems within our family and tarnished our *ie* image in the community. In February 2010, Yukie desperately contacted me for the first time in the United States, begging me to rescue her. I flew to Japan the next month and removed Yukie from the family house. Although already petite, she now weighed only 70 pounds. A few months later, I learned that she also had suffered severe *utsu* and bipolar disorder. She refused food and drink, begged me to let her die, and even asked me to kill her and to die alongside her. She turned into a complete stranger to me. No *utsu* medicine or treatment worked. She had stubbornly endured her abuse and fear for too long.

Without our family's love and support, it has been extremely difficult for me to take care of Yukie by myself. She requires constant attention and care, although she used to be such an independent, strong, confident woman. After four years under my care, Yukie has regained weight—up to 110 pounds now—and has discontinued constantly blaming herself. She no longer talks about committing suicide.

Conclusion

Utsu means "depression," but as a health issue in Japan, it means so much more. In women, when it is tied to the panopticon of *ie*, the risk of suicide, or even just suicidal thoughts—a prison of its own—increases, as the studies cited here show. Complicating matters, a good mother/wife and her family most likely will deny that she has *utsu*. I denied it, too, when my friends asked me if my mother had *utsu*. My mother is still in denial but accepts treatment. I know she is aware, however, because she blames herself for stigmatizing her family. That they also blame her depresses her further, which at one point caused her to refuse to eat, resulting in a severe weight loss that, though she has recovered, surely left her with profound health problems that may not yet be manifest. She also suffered from sleep deprivation. Her mind has been troubled continuously for the past four years; for a while, when she could, she claimed that she seldom slept, trying to compensate by working more and working harder, all of which served to stress her more and compound her depression. Suicide not only looked attractive, but also seemed the only option—hence her attempt to imitate *samurai*'s *hara-kiri* [suicide by cutting through the stomach].The very fact that sociable, vivacious Yukie would try to kill herself points to an aspect of *utsu* that further stigmatizes the patient and everyone around her: personality change. It can become extremely challenging for family members to take care of the *utsu* patient. Without sufficient knowledge of *utsu* and abundant patience, caretakers may easily misunderstand the *utsu* patient and mistreat her. Since family caretakers in Japan, under *ie*'s continuing influence, are always women, they may find themselves overburdened and susceptible to *utsu* themselves. What is needed is a good self-monitoring system—not the panopticon—and family and community support, not stigmatization.

In the panopticon of *ie* today, model prisoners—those who aspire to the highest ideals—employ the "unequal gaze" to seek to differentiate themselves from the rest. Both Akie and Yukie represent such model prisoners. They tried to become *alterity* through disciplining and punishing themselves according to the *ie* prescriptions. Yukie was proud of her wedding dowry, which her parents prepared, but little could she have known that she would not have much chance to wear her pretty dowry *kimono* at all in her married life (see Akita, 2009). In the *ie* panopticon, prisoners internalize the *ie* prescriptions. Akie and Yukie endured for the sake of *ie*. Akie complained only privately to her birth mother about having been given her away to her aunt's family. Yukie devoted her married life to caring for her husband, the children, and her mother-in-law until she died, and she found little time left over for her own family. Before going on an overseas trip, Yukie would work extra hard to weed the garden and make her house and yard look neat and clean so that no one in the neighborhood could criticize her or her family during her absence. Yukie had to take vacations secretly because she did not want her neighbors to think she was a lazy mother/wife. Yukie was always alert to the *ie* guards' gazes, especially the female guards' gazes.

While rescuing my mother in 2010, I was able to get some help from Akie's daughter, my cousin, whom I had not seen since Akie's funeral in 1998. My cousin told me for the first time in 2010 that Akie had developed *utsu* before she committed suicide. It takes years or sometimes is not even possible to learn such private information because it represents testimony against *ie*. My cousin held that secret close for 12 years because of the threat of stigma that others might inflict on Akie's high *ie* survivors, my cousin's maiden family. My cousin was the prisoner/guard observing her family with the unequal gaze.

Removing my mother from the family home also represented a rejection of *ie*, even though it was a matter of my mother's life and death. I have been punished severely by the unwritten law of *ie*; I am now shunned by my family, relatives, and the people in my former community. The panopticon of *ie* is run by men and women, but women prisoners and guards become better trained disciplinarians over generations. But I moved myself out of that dungeon long ago and developed critical thinking for myself through my education in the United States. I will never return to the prison of *ie*. I will continue to speak for the voiceless women who are imprisoned.

References

Akita, K. (2003). Critical ethnography of my aunt's suicide: Intergenerational family conflict in Japan. *Human Communication: A Journal of the Pacific and Asian Communication Association, 6*(1), 59–79.

Akita, K. (2005). *Interaction in the* Onnna-Yu: *The women's section of a bathhouse in Japan,* Unpublished Doctoral Dissertation, Athens, OH.

Akita, K. (2006). The professional suicide of a Japanese woman teacher. In W. Ashton & D. Denton (Eds.), *Spirituality, ethnography, and teaching* (pp. 56–71). New York: Peter Lang.

Akita, K. (2009). A story of *tansu*, a chest of drawers: Japanese women's love, hope, and despair. *Journal of Public and Private in Contemporary History,* No. 4, 17–33.

Bartholet, J. (1996, June 3). Silent princess. *Newsweek* (U.S. edition), p. 38.

Benedict, R. (1946). *The chrysanthemum and the sword: Patterns of Japanese culture.* Tokyo: Charles E. Tuttle.

Chandler, C., & Tsai, Y. (1993). Suicide in Japan and in the West: Evidence for Durkheim's theory. *International Journal of Comparative Sociology, 34*(3–4), 224–259.

Foucault, M. (1977). *Discipline and punish: The birth of the prison* (A. Sheridan, Trans.). New York: Vintage Books.

Goldstein-Gidoni, O. (1999). Kimono and the construction of gendered and cultural identity. *Ethnology, 38*(4), 351–370.

Gordon, M. (2011). Understanding Japanese society through life after death. *Japan Forum 23*(3), 363–383.

Hane, M. (1982). *Peasants, rebels, and outcastes: The underside of modern Japan.* New York: Pantheon Books.

Hirai, T. (2004). *Utsubyo no chiryo point* [Key points to treat *utsu*]. Osaka: Sogensha.

Inoue, H. (2000). *Hakao meguru kazoku ron: Dareto hairuka, darega mamoruka* [Family dispute over grave: Who wants to be buried with? Who has to maintain the grave?]. Tokyo: Heibonsha.

Inoue, M. (2006). *Vicarious language: Gender and linguistic modernity in Japan.* Berkeley: University of California Press.

Kano, M. (1983). *Senzen Ie no Shisou* [Ideology of Ie before WWII]. Tokyo: Sobunsha.

Kano, M. (1989). *Fujin, josei, onna: Joseishi no toi* [Ladies, women, female: Questions over women's history]. Tokyo: Iwanami shinsho.

Kano, M. (2007). *Kano Masanao, shisoushi ronshuu* [Kano Masanao's Ideology collection], *vol. 2.* Tokyo: Iwanami shinsho.

Kitanaka, J. (2012). Depression in Japan: Psychiatric cures for a society in distress. Princeton, NJ: Princeton University Press.

Kitche, S. (1995). Antecedents of the Japanese distribution system—Formative agents in Tokugawa Japan. *Japan and the World Economy, 7*(2), 199–210.

Kondo, D. (1990). *Crafting selves: Power, gender and discourses of identity in a Japanese workplace.* Chicago: University of Chicago Press.

Koyama, T. (1961). *The changing social position of women in Japan.* Geneva, Switzerland: Unesco.

Mihalopoulos, B. (2009). Mediating the good life: Prostitution and the Japanese woman's Christian Temperance Union, 1880s–1920s. *Gender and History, 21*(1), 19–38.

Ministry of Health, Labour and Welfare. (2011). Survey results on *utsu* patients. Tokyo: Ministry's Statistical Research Analysis Office.

Ministry of Health, Labour and Welfare. (2010). Survey results on *utsu* patients. Tokyo: Ministry's Statistical Research Analysis Office.

Nitobe, I. (1909). *Bushido, the soul of Japan: An exposition of Japanese thought.* New York: Knickerbocker Press.

Nolte, S., & Hastings, S. (1991). The Meiji state's policy toward women, 1890–1910. In G. Bernstein (Ed.), *Recreating Japanese women, 1600–1945* (pp. 151–174). Berkeley: University of California Press.

Ono, Y. (2000). *Utsu o naosu* [Healing utsu]. Tokyo: PHP Shinsho.

Parry, R. (2008, October 25). Sympathy turns to skepticism as courtiers whisper that princess does not do her duty. *The Times,* p. 47.

Plath, D. W. (1964). *The after hours: Modern Japan and the search for enjoyment.* Berkeley: University of California Press.

Plath, D. W. (1980). *Long engagements: Maturity in modern Japan.* Stanford, CA: Stanford University Press.

Robertson, J. (1991). The Shingaku woman: Straight from the heart. In G. L. Bernstein (Ed.), *Recreating Japanese women, 1600–1945* (pp. 88–107). Berkeley: University of California Press.

Ryall, J. (2008, June 18). Ailing Japanese princess losing support of public. *South China Morning Post,* p. 11.

Ryall, J. (2012, December 10). Japan's Crown Princess Masako discusses her illness on 49th birthday; Crown Princess Masako, the wife of the heir to the Japanese throne, marked her 49th birthday on Sunday apologising for being ill and absent from public life for so many years. *The Telegraph.* Retrieved January 29, 2013, at telegraph.co.uk.

Shimozono, S. (2004). *Utsu karano dasshutsu* [Exit from *utsu*]. Tokyo: Nihon hyoron sha.

Takayama, H. (2001, August 27). Japan's crowning dream. *Atlantic Edition,* p. 47.

Taussig, M. (1993). *Mimesis and alterity: A particular history of the senses.* New York: Routledge.

Tonomura, H. (1999). Sexual violence against women: Legal and extralegal treatment in premodern warrior societies. In H. Tonomura, A. Walthall, & H. Wakita (Eds.), *Women and class in Japanese history* (pp. 135–152). Ann Arbor: University of Michigan.

United Nations Department of Economic and Social Affairs. (2011). *World population prospects, the 2010 revision.*

Section IV

Sex, Sexuality, Relational Health, and Womanhood

9 Sexual and Relational Health Messages for Women Who Have Sex with Women

Sandra L. Faulkner, Andrea M. Davis, Manda V. Hicks and Pamela J. Lannutti

Introduction

Although much attention has been paid to sexual risk and negotiation of sexual risk-reducing behaviors between women and their male partners, less research has been done on sexual health communication aimed at or engaged in by women who have sex with women (WSW) (Bailey, Farquhar, Owen, & Mangtani, 2004; Feathers, Marks, Mindel, & Estcourt, 2000). There is a misconception among WSW, and the public in general, that WSW's relatively low rates of sexually transmitted infections (STIs) and low risk for STI transmission from female-to-female sexual contact make it less necessary to address safer sex practices among WSW. In fact, WSW are still at risk for many STIs, bacterial, viral, and protozoal infections that have long-term health consequences, such as human papillomavirus (HPV), which can be easily transmitted through female-to-female sexual contact (CDC, 2012). Further, most WSW have either a history or current practice of having sex with men; 53% to 99% of WSW in one study reported having had sex with men and had plans to continue the practice in the future, therefore increasing their risk of STI contraction and transmission beyond what would be expected of a woman who has sex exclusively with women (Diamant, Schuster, McGuigan, et al., 1999). More specifically, there is a need to prioritize sexual health as it is framed by cultural, political, and relational factors—in other words, observing how sexual health is framed within the dominant discourse. To this end, we use standpoint theory to frame data from an online survey and a content analysis of sexuality texts targeted at WSW. This research gives voice to how WSW communicate with their peers, partners, and healthcare providers about sexuality.

WSW and Safer Sex

Research on women and sexual risk-reducing behaviors has shown that relational factors, such as trust and partner face-saving, have influenced negotiation of safer sex behavior (Civic, 2000; Faulkner & Mansfield, 2002). Thus, we focus on sexual health messages in the wider context of relationships, not only on the medical and sexual practice information in the messages, but also on communication (e.g., self-disclosure) and relational (e.g., relationship goals and consequences) aspects of sexual health messages. Sexual health consists of a state of physical, mental, and social well-being related to one's sexuality and necessitates positivity and respect for sexuality and sexual relationships that are pleasurable, safe, and free from coercion, discrimination, and violence (WHO, 2012). Considering one's self to not be at risk for STIs is based in large part on faulty perception; and faulty perceptions are the result of a dominant discourse that does not include the circumstances of all real lived lives. Dolan's (2005) study on lesbian women and sexual health revealed institutional, interpersonal, circumstantial, and labeling barriers to the construction of risk and vulnerability. Participants did not receive information on safer sex for WSW from private doctors or school-based sex education programs, often remained closeted with healthcare providers, considered themselves at low risk for STIs, even if engaging in risky behavior, and found it difficult to talk about STIs with partners.

Although WSW who have never had sex with men have low rates of STIs (Robers et al., 2000), most women who identify as lesbian or bisexual have had heterosexual intercourse, thereby raising their STI risk (Koh, 2000). Scheer et al. (2002) determined that the WSW population that included women who had sex with men "were significantly more likely to report past and recent high-risk sexual behavior" (p. 1111). Indeed, Scheer et al. (2002) claim that women who have had sex with men and women potentially face a higher risk of STIs than do women who have sex only with men or only with women. Several studies argue that WSW do not have high rates of self-reported safer sex practices (Dolan, 2005; Morrow & Allsworth, 2000). Dolan and Davis (2003) found that some lesbian women did not consider themselves at risk for STIs because of their identity and sexual practices as lesbians, but more participants in this study felt they were safe as a result of "social inoculation"—the concept that because of their "social circle's selectivity, lesbian women enjoy conditional protections against infections and other sexual health problems" (p. 31).

Research suggests that WSW do not access healthcare to the extent heterosexual women do and that those women who do receive healthcare are not always forthcoming about their sexual orientation (Trippett & Bain, 1992). This lack of healthcare might relate both to the level to which WSW are educated about sexual risk and to the degree to which they know of safer sex options, particularly as relating to sex with other women. It seems then that public discourse represents struggles with an adequate conceptualization of WSW and an identification of their particular health needs and risk behaviors.

WSW and Relational Health

Research comparing the relational qualities and satisfaction correlates for different-sex and same-sex couples has shown that the experiences of these couple types are more similar than different (see Kurdek, 2005, for review). However, the differences among different-sex and same-sex couples that do exist have been shown to have a significant impact on the quality of same-sex couples. Specifically, same-sex couples are vulnerable to the negative effects of social stigma, resulting in sexual minority stress, lack of familial support of the couple, and restrictions in legal relationship recognition and protection (Kurdek, 2005; Mohr & Daly, 2008; Riggle, Rostosky, & Horne, 2010). Female–female couples may differ from male–male couples in that female–female couples are vulnerable to the effects of sexism as well as sexual orientation stigma (Slater, 1995). Studies of relational satisfaction among female–female couples suggest that to understand the relational health of WSW's relationships, it is important to consider sexual orientation-related factors, such as stigma, internalized homophobia, and degree of "outness" (Beals & Peplau, 2001; Beals, Impett, & Peplau, 2002). These factors contribute to the unique standpoint of WSW. Thus, when considering the sexual and relational health of WSW, it is important to acknowledge the uniqueness of their romantic relationships.

Feminist Standpoint Theory

Feminist standpoint theory recognizes that knowledge takes place in particular contexts and that knowledge and accounts of knowledge are neither neutral nor universal. Yet the theorizing and experiences of some groups have not counted as knowledge in Western culture (Harding, 2004). Feminist standpoint theory is important in the study of WSW because inaccurate and incomplete knowledge accompanies any sexual behavior that does not fit neatly into the existing dominant culture. Early feminist standpoint theories pointed out the dubious connection between the dominant culture and the theories it produced and argued that a position of power and privilege serves as the invisible center of knowledge production.

Collins (1986) presents the same argument, stating that some members of a society are afforded a greater vantage point than others (and themselves) precisely because of extreme discrepancies in power and privilege. What remains "invisible and taken for granted by those in power becomes clear to those who witness all the effort that goes into naturalizing supremacy and oppression" (Hicks, 2011, p. 36). The lives and practices of WSW offer an opportunity to achieve a standpoint that is mindful and reflective of realities otherwise marginalized or absent within the dominant discourse, thereby making space in the world of sexual possibilities for more truths rather than one truth.

Overall, standpoint theorists argue that a particular privileged view of the world serves as the allegedly neutral center from which knowledge is produced and that center is typically not representative of a diversity of lived experiences. Experiences differ significantly depending on one's relation to privilege. The understandings of those not situated as the recipients of privileged race, gender, normative understandings of sexual identity, or other privilege will differ in systematic ways from those with privilege. Drawing on their own experiences and theorizing, groups outside the mainstream work toward self-valuation and self-determination to achieve a standpoint. Meanwhile, what is assumed to be a neutral or universal perspective is often the standpoint of dominant groups. This standpoint is reflected in the dominant discourse and serves to limit or exclude the perspectives of those whose lived experiences are not affirmed within the dominant culture. The concept that sexuality is fluid, or that individuals conduct their sexual lives in a way that is not recognizable within the dominant discourse, tends to threaten or confuse the status quo (Warner, 1999) and to limit the potentialities of the marginalized by only providing one position within the discourse (Edelman, 2004).

Standpoint epistemology is useful because it encourages us to denaturalize positions often seen as neutral and therefore apolitical. It allows us to see such privileged positions as existing among many others. Therefore, our research identifies how relationship issues, sexual health, and sexuality are portrayed in sexuality texts and examines how the complexity of WSW's sexuality is constructed and negotiated within dominant discourse. The following questions guided our research: (1) What dominant and marginalized sexual health and relational health messages are represented in sexuality books targeted to WSW?; (2) what considerations influence safer sexual practices among WSW?; and (3) how do WSW perceive talk about sex and sexuality with friends? with partners? with healthcare providers?

Content Analysis of Sexuality Texts/Survey with WSW

Our qualitative content coding of sexual education messages revealed that some messages negotiated the complexity of discourses related to sex and relationships, whereas others strengthened problematic barriers to safe sexual and relational choices (Faulkner, Davis, Hicks, & Lannutti, 2011). Put differently, some messages both acknowledged and challenged the dominant discourse, whereas others simply functioned within its assumptions. We used qualitative content analysis to reveal textual content themes that address sexual advice within sexuality texts targeted to WSW (Lindlof & Taylor, 2010). The texts we examined are marked with an asterisk in the References section. We choose to focus on messages found in books about sex between women because they represent an important source of information for WSW (Pecoskie, 2005). We also conducted a complementary online survey with WSW (Faulkner & Lannutti, 2012). The survey questions focused on what conversations WSW are having and how they feel about these conversations. Participants were recruited by online snowball sampling and through researchers' friend networks online. A total of 144 females completed the survey: 110 identified as lesbian, 18 as bisexual, 1 as questioning, 1 as straight, and 14 as other; 4 did not report their orientation. Ages ranged from 20 to 63 years of age, with an average age of 33 years. Three participants reported being of mixed racial background, 119 identified as white, 3 Asian, 10 African American, 1 Mexican American, 2 Jewish, 2 Latina, and 1 Chicano; 10 did not report their racial background.

Sexual and Relational Health Themes

We present the themes from the content analyses and follow with findings from the survey study to compare and contrast our analysis of texts with WSW's voices about sexual and relational health.

Partner Talk

All of the texts stated the importance of good communication between partners in multiple areas of the relationship. Good communication was defined as requiring partner trust, sensitivity to conversational contexts, curiosity, openness, honesty, and willingness and ability to negotiate. Because of the (often) emotional context involved in discussions about sex, removing sexual tension and personal judgments through the choice of setting and planning what to talk about can make the conversation easier and more productive.

Authors discussed talk with a partner as a sexual health behavior that meant discussion of risk, sexual history, and sexual behaviors. "Get tested, and talk with her about her body too. It's not a crime to have a sexually transmitted disease, but they are zero fun, and some have serious consequences" (Cage, 2004, p. 29). All texts emphasized that timing and planning were important. Most of the texts emphasized that discussing risky behaviors gives partners the information to decide what the best options are for minimizing future risk. Sexual behaviors were noted to be risky emotionally and physically; therefore, talk with a partner needed to be negotiated.

Although text authors promote the importance of partner talk in WSW's sexual health, WSW who completed our survey indicated overall desire to talk with their partners about sex openly and honestly, though many respondents described the difficulties with doing so. In the survey, we asked WSW about discussions with new partners and long-term partners regarding STI risk, safer sex strategies, and sexual history. Most of the women (81.6%) indicated that they discussed STI risk with new partners, and a majority (75%) indicated that they discussed safer sex strategies with new partners. Fewer women (69.5%) said they discussed STI risk or safer sex (63.1%) with long-term partners, perhaps because this seemed less important in a long-term relationship. Women (61.1%) indicated that talking about *safer sex strategies* with a partner was uncomfortable. However, more than half of the women (62.1%) said talking about their *sexual history* with a partner was not uncomfortable.

Survey participants explained a variety of problems that occurred when sexual partners discussed STI risk, sexual history, and safer sex. The themes that emerged from these responses were: (1) the other person created a negative climate, (2) one or both partners tried to avoid discussing it, (3) there was lack of honesty in conversations, (4) a feeling of shame or embarrassment emerged, (5) some partners were naïve, and (6) timing or situational factors arose.

Social Networks

Our content analysis revealed that authors discussed social networks as both a positive and negative aspect of the WSW community. "Lesbians' historical reticence and nervousness about talking about sex has been exacerbated by the bitter debates within lesbian sexual politics. Who wanted to risk being denounced, excommunicated from the lesbian club, labeled a terrible person because she talked openly?" (O'Sullivan & Parmar, 1992, p. 37). The influences of WSW's social networks were more often described by authors as helpful rather than harmful. The small networks of WSW, particularly the small dating pools among some friends, are noted in these texts as a source of irritation at times. On a more positive note, social networks were viewed as a way to combat heterosexism in other facets of WSWs' daily lives. Even with supportive heterosexual friends, it is often hard to explain the challenges of being nonheterosexual. Social networks for WSW made up of other WSW can help alleviate the expectations of a heterosexist, mainstream society. A community was also important for asking sexual health and pleasure questions that WSW could not ask a healthcare provider.

WSW who participated in our survey also discussed the influence of social networks in WSWs' sexual and relational health. Participants explained how they discussed sex and sexuality with their friends who had sex with women. Three themes emerged from their responses: (1) open, honest, or often, (2) do not or rarely discuss, and (3) some topics discussed while others not. Participants overwhelmingly fell into two opposing groups—those who openly discussed sex and sexuality with their friends (31 responses) and those who did not (30 responses).

Participants explained that they discussed some topics about sex and sexuality while avoiding others. Women differentiated between sex and sexuality and indicated that they discussed sexuality but not sex or safer sex acts. For example, "I don't discuss sexual activity but do discuss sexuality. It is usually in the context of identity development, social interaction, youth development, and school environment/threat for LGBTIQ individuals." Some women were interested in sharing their knowledge with others, especially those who were at risk, less educated, or younger. They felt that younger women were taking more risks and needed to be informed: "Hooking up seems to be the norm these days. I make sure the younger baby dykes protect themselves when trolling for late night love."

Thus, like text authors, participants in our survey saw the potential of social networks to be beneficial for WSW sexual and relational health, but also indicated that the community needed more resources and different social norms around sexual and relational health. In the survey, women provided several suggestions on how to get WSW to engage more frequently in safer sex practices. Participants believed that having more research conducted in the WSW community, making statistics available to the WSW community, and having mediated campaigns, advertisements, media portrayals, and education for both the community and healthcare providers would be beneficial and encourage WSW to engage in safer sex practices. Within WSW communities, participants believed that having more lighthearted and open conversations and norm setting within the community would also be beneficial. Finally, barriers should be more appealing, easier to access and distributed more widely, and safer sex should be eroticized.

Sexual Health

In many of the texts we examined in our content analysis, deconstruction of the dominant discourse was seen as necessary for crafting effective sexual health messages. For example, Newman (2004) writes that "[y]ou may believe that because you're in a committed monogamous relationship you're exempt from safer-sex concerns. If that were true, there would be far fewer of us with herpes and HPV" (pp. 69–70). Newman's observation demonstrates an achieved standpoint; one that recognizes the dominant discourse and challenges its assumptions. This quote provides a clear example of how most of the texts deconstructed false perceptions of safety: Monogamous individuals have sexual risk owing to past relationships (monogamous and nonmonogamous) as well as the level of individuals' honesty. The perception of lower risk in the WSW community exists because of the often-quoted research that WSW have lower STI transmission rates than heterosexual women. Several authors argued that most WSW have, in fact, also had sex with men, thus negating any lessened STI risk.

HIV and STIs were discussed from historical perspectives, both social histories and personal histories. Some of the claims were informative, apparently directed at those who didn't know the history of HIV/AIDS, or at least didn't know the role of lesbians in the history of HIV/AIDS. O'Sullivan and Parmar (1992) state further that individuals who are from lower socioeconomic classes are often labeled as "agents of their own sickness" (p. 14), deserving blame for being infected, therefore showing HIV/AIDS separate from middle-class individuals. The texts attempt to put sexual messages in a historical context, suggesting that from this perspective, sex is more than coupling—it is an understanding of the sociohistorical forces that shape (and force) sexuality and sexual behavior.

The authors also emphasize the role of personal sexual history in relation to HIV/STIs. Cage (2004), in a section labeled "Which STDs Do Lesbians Really Need to Know About." discusses HPV, Chlamydia, and HIV, among others. She indicates that although several STIs are perceived to influence heterosexual women more than lesbian women, "Many lesbian-identified women weren't always, and unfortunately sometimes the past comes back to haunt you" (p. 234). Here Cage draws the reader's attention to the difference between identity and behavior, suggesting that the labels and categories that exist in the dominant discourse do not always accurately reflect the lived experiences behind them. Bright (1998) attempts to incite readers: "We have now reached a point, because of AIDS, where we either confront our taboos and get real, or we're going to watch our own silence and secrecy kill us" (Bright, 1998, p. 135). At the same time, Bright (1998) emphasizes that lesbians need to "own up to AIDS' effect on our lives" (p. 130) and describes how the details of safer sexual practice can distract: "The real dilemma of women's sexuality and AIDS is fear, stigma, humiliation, and estrangement. The goal is to feel close, sexy and passionate—and turn on and dig yourself" (p. 133).

Most of the texts noted the importance of WSW getting regular sexual health check-ups and acknowledged that many WSW do not get check-ups because they are uncomfortable with the process or the physician. "Your physician may downplay your concerns about your sex life. She may feel uncomfortable talking to you about sex between women. ... Your physician may view lesbians as not sexually "active"—since they presume you're not having sex with men (Newman, 2004, pp. 35–36)." Even when WSW do get check-ups, they may have care providers who are inexperienced and uncomfortable working with non-heterosexual women. Thus, they often do not receive adequate care. Bright (1998), for instance, described a hands-on fisting workshop she led that included a demonstration and a question and answer session. "This is simply something you can't ask your doctor, not only because you're embarrassed, but because the damn doctor doesn't know anything about it!" (pp. 80–81). Bright reminds WSW that there are sexual practices outside of the assumptions of dominant cultural sexual practices and their accompanying medical authority. Stevens and Wunder (2002) encouraged readers to take the initiative and ask friends for references, consult local LGBT papers, and/or do phone interviews to determine if a care provider was a good fit. The implicit message is that learning what one needs and finding out how to secure these needs are ways to redefine agency in healthcare.

Authors often used WSW's narratives to emphasize that barriers to practicing safer sex can be overcome and be replaced with motivation to engage in safer sexual behaviors. Examples used in texts to demonstrate the perception of safer sex as inconvenient, stifling, and unattractive are inaccurate. In fact, safer sex allows WSW to engage in a wider variety of sexual behaviors (Stevens & Wunder, 2002).

When asked about what types of conversations they have had with health-care providers about sex, sexuality, and health, the survey respondents over-whelmingly mentioned the amount of talk they have with their providers. Conversations ranged from none to minimal to very open and honest, with most having no or limited conversations with healthcare providers. Some of the women felt embarrassed or uncomfortable discussing sexual topics with their healthcare providers. For instance, one woman explained, "Most of my healthcare providers have asked about my sexual orientation, and I've disclosed to them. Beyond that, I'm always amazed at how few ask any questions about my actual sexual behavior—and how uncomfortable I feel asking them questions, even though I'm comfortable with the subject." Other women explained they had very minimal discussions with their healthcare providers or that providers only knew their sexual orientation. For example, "My doctors are aware of my orientation and seem nonjudgmental. They do not ask any specific questions, other than the standard 'Is there abuse in your home? Do you feel safe?' I have never had a specific sexual issue that I have asked a doctor about. Since I am open with my doctors, I do not know how this compares with questions that they might ask their straight patients."

Because of the overwhelming lack of in-depth conversations, it is no surprise that many of the women were disappointed with the care they received, the knowledge of healthcare providers about lesbian sex issues, and their preoccupation with pregnancy. Another woman expressed her concern by stating: "I think the medical system leaves a lot to be desired, which is why I don't use it. Though I must say that the old "Do you have sex?" "Yes," "What kind of birth control do you use?" "None" conversation has happened several times to me, and I think that it's idiotic every single time. That conversation should go, "Do you have sex with men?" "No," and so on. Despite the dissatisfaction, many of the women did mention at least some discussion about STIs/HIV, protection, and safer sex concerns, but the responses they received were not always what they were hoping for. Not all of the healthcare providers were well versed in safer sex prac-tices for lesbian women. For instance, one woman said they had "no real conversations on safe sex in terms of barriers, etc. (I felt like I knew more than they did to be honest when it came to lesbian sex practices)." Finally, a few of the women mentioned specifically seeking out female, lesbian, or LBGTQ-friendly healthcare providers. Although this is not always possible because of location and insurance or healthcare issues, these women did seem to be more satisfied with the care they received."

Conclusion

Our research demonstrates the complexity of crafting sexual and relational health messages for WSW. The relational and sexual health messages found in the sexuality texts demonstrate the competing discourses that must be negotiated in order to make the sexual lives and sexual health of WSW intelligible as women in the survey indicated. The texts represent one type of effort to combat the invisibility of WSW sexual health risk and assist WSW in making healthier sexual and relational choices. Even as such, our analysis demonstrates the ways in which some messages may strengthen problematic barriers to safe sexual and relational choices. The study highlights the need to engage in competing discourses when crafting effective sexual health messages and identifying productive interventions.

The emphasis on knowing one's own body, exploring one's desire and pleasure, being conscious of identities and the role of social networks, and especially talking to partners about sexual pleasure and desire contrasted with discourse of WSW's sexual shame, invisibility, and silence. Through the use of individual and coupled women's stories, including the authors' stories, these texts contended with the competition between discourses by giving voice to marginalized discourses in a polemical-transformative struggle. That is, the voicing of marginal discourses of relational identities and behaviors are set against dominant ideas of static notions of identity and conceptualizations of WSW's sexuality to ultimately transform WSW's sexuality and provide new meaning, a discursive transformation.

This inquiry into sexual and relational health messages directed at WSW demarcated the particular standpoint of WSW. That is, the assumptions, expectations, and innovations surrounding WSW's sexual health and identity are revealed in this particular negotiation of self and sexual expression. The use of personal narratives from authors and the WSW community establish standpoints. The dominant discourse is pervasive, though many texts gave voice to marginal discourses. A recurring theme/sentence in some texts was that lesbian identity is rigid and shamed by sex with men. This indicates one barrier to sexual health that needs to be addressed: WSW should be reminded that their entire sexual history matters. One strategy for contending with the stigmatization of sex with men is to acknowledge that people don't always have sex with the same object of desire (Sedgwick, 2008).

Another barrier to sexual and relational health that should be addressed is the association of pleasure with sexual health. Some of the texts made the association explicit. Once WSW see safer sex represented in dominant discourse, it may be easier to incorporate it into our own lives. The complex messages that WSW's sexuality and desire are different from the dominant representations, that it is multilayered, and that individuals do not all arrive in the same manner, makes the strategy of pairing safer sex practices with sexual pleasure important. The "condoms are a drag" discourse competes with other methods/practices feeding into the larger heteronormative discourse that sex should occur within the safety of married monogamy. Anything that indicates otherwise damages notions of good sex.

The findings from this research demonstrate the importance of engaging competing discourses when crafting effective sexual health messages and identifying productive interventions. When sexual identities or sexual behaviors marked as unintelligible or "deviant" make their way into the public discourse, a great deal of negotiation and management of meaning is necessary. These new perspectives represent achieved standpoints wherein traditional ways of understanding and experiencing the world are expanded. According to Harding (2004), a feminist standpoint perspective provides "a source of critical insight about how the dominant society thinks and is structured" (p. 7). Therefore, these new standpoints alert us to underlying assumptions about sexuality that are challenged or altered in the process of creating new knowledge.

Power, McNair, and Carr (2009) argue that WSW are excluded from the dominant sexual discourse that informs safer sex practice. The current study demonstrates the ways that multiple and competing discourses are manifested in some safer sex and relational health messages aimed at WSW. Future studies should examine the relational and sexual health messages in other forms of media. Further, sexual and relational health messages among WSW and between WSW and their healthcare providers should be further analyzed with the goal of finding ways to create effective sexual health messages for WSW and raise awareness about the sexual health risks and needs of WSW among WSW and healthcare providers.

References

Bailey, J. V., Farquhar, C., Owen, C., & Mangtani, P. (2004). Sexually transmitted infections in women who have sex with women. *Sexually Transmitted Infections, 80*, 244–246. doi:10.1136/sti.2003.007641.

Beals, K. P., Impett, E. A., & Peplau, L. A. (2002). Lesbians in love: Why some relationships endure and others end. *Journal of Lesbian Studies, 6*, 53–63.

Beals, K. P., & Peplau, L. A. (2001). Social involvement, disclosure of sexual orientation, and the quality of lesbian relationships. *Psychology of Women Quarterly, 25*, 10–19.

Bright, S. (1998). *Susie Sexpert's lesbian sex world* (2nd ed.) San Francisco: Cleis Press.

Cage, D. (Ed) (2004). *On our backs guide to lesbian sex.* Los Angeles: Alyson Press.

Carpenter, L. M. (2002). Analyzing textual material. In M. W. Wiederman & B. E. Whitley Jr. (Eds.), *Handbook for conducting research on human sexuality* (pp. 327–343). Mahwah, NJ: Erlbaum.

Centers for Disease Control. (2012). CDC fact sheet: HIV/AIDS among women who have sex with women. Available at http://www.cdc.gov/lgbthealth/women.htm.

Civic, D. (2000). College students' reason for the nonuse of condoms within dating relationships. *Journal of Sex and Marital Therapy, 26*, 95–105. doi:10.1080/009262300278678.

Collins, P. H. (1986). Learning from the outsider within: The sociological significance of Black feminist thought. *Social Problems, 33*(6), S14–S32. Retrieved from http://ucpressjournals.com/journal.asp?j=sp.

Diamant, A. L., Schuster M. A., McGuigan, K., et al. (1999). Lesbians' sexual history with men: Implications for taking a sexual history. *Archives of Internal Medicine, 159*, 2730–2736.

Dolan, K. A. (2005). Lesbian women and sexual health: The social construction of risk and susceptibility. New York: Haworth Press.

Dolan, K. A., & Davis, P. W. (2003). HIV testing among lesbian women: Social contexts and subjective meanings. *Journal of Homosexuality, 54*(3), 307–324.

Edelman, L. (2004). *No future: Queer theory and the death drive*. Durham, NC: Duke University Press.

Faulkner, S. L., Davis, A. M., Hicks, M. V., & Lannutti, P. J. (2011, November). A content analysis of sexual and relational health messages for women who have sex with women. Paper presentation at the annual meeting of the National Communication Association, New Orleans, LA.

Faulkner, S. L., & Lannutti, P. J. (2012, July). WSW (women who have sex with women) and sexual talk with family, friends, and healthcare providers: A pilot study. Panel presentation at the biannual meeting of the International Association of Relationship Research, Chicago.

Faulkner, S. L., & Mansfield, P. K. (2002). Reconciling messages: The process of sexual talk for Latinas. *Qualitative Health Research, 12*, 310–328.

Feathers, K., Marks, C., Mindel, A., & Estcourt, C. S. (2000). Sexually transmitted infections and risk behaviors in women who have sex with women. *Sexually Transmitted Infections, 76*, 345–349. doi:10.1136/sti.76.5.345.

Fishman, S. J., & Anderson, E. H. (2003). Perception of HIV and safer sexual behaviors among lesbians. *Journal of the Association of Nurses in AIDS Care, 14*(6), 48–55. doi:10.1016/S1055-3290(05)60068-4.

Harding, S. (2004). Introduction: Standpoint theory as a site of political, philosophic, and scientific debate. In Sandra Harding (Ed.), *The feminist standpoint theory reader: Intellectual and political controversies* (1–15). New York: Routledge.

Hicks, M. V. (2011). Negotiating gendered expectations: The basic social processes of women in the military (Unpublished doctoral dissertation). Bowling Green State University, Ohio. Retrieved from https://etd.ohiolink.edu/ap/10?0::NO:10:P10_ACCESSION_NUM: bgsu1319580341.

Koh, A. S. (2000). Use of preventive health behaviours by lesbian, bisexual and heterosexual women: Questionnaire survey. *Western Journal of Medicine, 172*, 379–387. Retrieved from http://group.bmj.com/products/journals.

Kurdek, L. A. (2005). What do we know about gay and lesbian couples? *Current Directions in Psychological Science, 14*, 251–254.

Lindlof, T. R., & Taylor, B. C. (2010). *Qualitative communication research methods* (3rd ed.). Thousand Oaks, CA: Sage.

McDaniel, J. (1995). *The lesbian couples' guide: Finding the right woman and creating a life together*. New York: Harper Perennial.

Mohr, J. J., & Daly, C. A. (2008). Sexual minority stress and changes in relationship quality in same-sex couples. *Journal of Social and Personal Relationships, 25*, 989–1007.

Morrow, K. M., & Allsworth, J. E. (2000). Sexual risk in lesbians and bisexual women. *Journal of the Gay and Lesbian Medical Association, 4*, 159–165. doi:10.1023/A:1026507721501.

Newman, F. (2004). *The whole lesbian sex book: A passionate guide for all of us* (2nd ed.). San Francisco: Cleis Press.

O'Sullivan, S. & Parmar, P. (1992). *Lesbians talk (safer) sex*. London: Scarlett Press.

Pecoskie, J. L. (2005). The intersection of "community" within the reading experience: Lesbian women's reflections on the book as text and object. *Canadian Journal of Information and Library Science, 29*(3), 335–349.

Power, J., McNair, R., & Carr, S. (2009). Absent sexual scripts: Lesbian and bisexual women's knowledge, attitudes, and action regarding safer sex and sexual health information. *Culture, Health, and Sexuality, 11,* 67–81. doi:10.1080/13691050802541674.

Riggle, E. D. B., Rostosky, S. S., & Horne, S. G. (2010). Psychological distress, well-being, and legal recognition in same-sex couples relationships. *Journal of Family Psychology, 24,* 82–86.

Robers, S. J., et al. (2000). Sexual behaviors and STDs of lesbians: Results of the Boston lesbian health project. *Journal of Lesbian Studies, 4*(3), 49–70. doi:10.1300/J155v04n03_03.

Rusbult, C. E. (1983). A longitudinal test of the investment model: The development (and deterioration) of satisfaction and commitment in heterosexual involvements. *Journal of Personality and Social Psychology, 45,* 101–117.

Scheer, S., Peterson, I., Page-Shafer, K., Delgado, V., Gleghorn, A., Ruiz, J., et al. (2002). Sexual and drug use behavior among women who have sex with both women and men: Results of a population-based survey. *American Journal of Public Health, 92,* 1110–1112. Retrieved from http://ajph.aphapublications.org.

Schulte, C. (2005). *Tantric sex for women: A guide for lesbian, bi, hetero, and solo lovers*. Alameda, CA: Hunter House.

Sedgwick. E. K. (2008). *Epistemology of the closet*. Berkeley: University of California Press.

Sincero, J. (2005). *The straight girls' guide to sleeping with chicks*. New York: Simon & Schuster.

Slater, S. (1995). The lesbian family life cycle: A contextual approach. *American Journal of Orthopsychiatry, 61,* 372–383.

Stevens, T., & Wunder, K. (2002). *Lesbian sex tips. A guide for anyone who wants to bring pleasure to the woman she (or he) loves*. Asheville, NC: Amazing Dreams Publishing.

Trippet, S. E., & Bain, J., (1992). Reasons American lesbians fail to seek traditional health care. *Health Care for Women International, 13,* 145–153. doi:10.1080/07399339209515987.

Warner, M. (1999). *The trouble with normal: Sex, politics, and the ethics of queer life*. New York: Free Press.

WHO (World Health Organization). (2012). Health topics: Sexual health. Retrieved from http://www.who.int/topics/sexual_health/en.

10 "Does this Mean I'm Dirty?"

The Complexities of Choice in Women's Conversations about HPV Vaccinations

Jennifer Malkowski

I stare intensely at the ceiling, counting the white particleboard squares separated by aluminum strips if only to avoid fixating on the fluorescent light overhead.

"Breathe." The nurse next to me is stroking my left hand, evaluating my comfort with worried eyes, and attempting to lend me her smile.

I pass and instead tense my jaw and mentally take out my frustration on a water stain inflicting an overhead square. I can barely see the doctor beyond my gowned, spread knees and look to the nurse for affirmation that I can and should be pissed that he is talking directly to my cervix:

Something, something, "I'm going to touch here," something, "it's very aggressive," something, something, "so young."

At this moment, I do not mind that his thick Indian accent disguises a cruel diagnostic play-by-play. I had to skip lacrosse practice to be here; I had to borrow my mom's car to get here; I am alone here.

"This is going to be cold," something, something, "hurts a little:" and with that, the chilly metal object slides into me and begins to over-turn an unseen dial. In my mind's eye I picture a woman's elegant scarf laying flat on a hard, slick surface and watch the doctor's hand find its center and begin to twist, twist so long and so steadily that each of the scarf's corners pull towards the center until it becomes contorted beyond elegance and beyond repair. I try and maintain the facade of familiarity with this type of procedure and this type of pain by nodding on cue and only weeping on the inside as if both exude maturity beyond my years, like I understood these risks before I wasted my time on that asshole. My hope is to avoid a condescending lecture.

No. No lectures. Not here, not now. Do not tell me that "I need to respect my body," do not tell me that "this is serious," do not tell me that "I am lucky" in any way. Shame on you. I already know I deserve this.

* * *

When I was 16 years old, I tested positive for a high-risk strain of human papillomavirus (HPV). To care for the condition, I followed the doctor's orders and underwent some rigorous and painful treatments. At the time, I was not informed about the nature of HPV or how I might have been exposed to the virus in the first place. Most significantly, I left the doctor's office unclear about what an HPV-positive status meant for my future sexual health. For the next two years, every three months I returned for an exam. For the next two years each report came back "clean." For the next decade I remained uncertain about how to disclose my HPV status to future sexual partners. What did a "clean" HPV-positive diagnosis mean for sexually responsible behavior? My personal coping mechanism often led me to abstain from sexual activity altogether to avoid having to reconcile my communication and identity dilemmas.

Many years after my initial diagnosis, a public health awareness campaign was launched and urged me to "tell someone" about the link between HPV and cervical cancer, a link that I had not known about despite my HPV-positive diagnosis. The advertisements did not mention the sexual nature of transmission nor male contribution to the problem and thus implicitly suggested some ground rules for discussion: I could talk about HPV in terms of cancer, but I should still remain silent about its classification as a sexually transmitted disease. On a personal level, this silence implied stigma and thus my abstinence from disclosure in the public arena continued. However, what the public health campaign did contribute to was a desire to find others who shared my silence.

In June 2006 the approval of GARDASIL®, a vaccine that blocks infection by four strains of the HPV virus, became of interest to public health agencies, political institutions, and advocacy organizations that recognize these strains as the cause of 70% of all cases of cervical cancer, and 90% of all cases of genital warts (Calloway, Jorgensen, Saraiya, & Tsui, 2006; CDC, 2006). Merck's next wave of advertising, dubbed "One Less," introduced the vaccine as the method for ensuring that each vaccinated girl would become "one less" cancer victim (Dederer, 2007). The campaign urged women to "tell someone" about how to become "one less" cancer victim, but implicitly added to the ground rules for HPV-related discussions. It was now acceptable to communicate about HPV in terms of cancer prevention, but the correlation between "responsibile" behavior and "consequences" largely dictated the tenor of those conversations. That is, the new medical vaccination technology provided women with an opportunity to proactively intervene and protect themselves if they elected to take medical action. Subsequently, if individual women decided not to heed the advice of medical professionals to get vaccinated and share their HPV knowledge with others, then, at least in part, an HPV-positive status implied a connection between "irresponsible" behavior and "deserved consequences." Understanding how women successfully communicated about HPV status in lieu of these implied rules and obligations emerged as a pressing issue among health scholars, professionals, and advocates invested in processes of disease intervention and prevention.

In an attempt to fully understand what types of discussions women have about HPV, the HPV vaccine, and their decision to become vaccinated, this chapter incorporates stories of positive HPV diagnoses, stories of "telling someone"—in this case, "telling other women"—about HPV and the HPV vaccination, and stories of testing negative for HPV in order to illuminate how women communicate about their health options. Specifically, I gathered data using focus groups, narrative interviews, and participant observation. Using women's own words, I have woven together three specific scenes that each interview worked to build. To do so, I read and reread the transcripts in order to allow the words of the participants to interact with each other in ways that revealed patterns about the factors that women consider with regard to this specific health option.

In the pages that follow, I explore the kinds of factors women communicate as influencing their decisions about health options and the specific concerns women communicate regarding the HPV vaccination. Specifically, I retell other women's stories that were prompted by the process of "telling others" about my condition. To better "balance rhetorical sources of creativity with the inevitable sources of rhetorical constraint" (Goodall, 2000, p. 92), their stories are told from beginning to end as if they were gathered during one focus group interview in which all of the women dialogued in the presence of one another. Both the presentation of the data in this manner and the patterns illuminated therein ought to complicate and deconstruct the notion of "choice" surrounding HPV prevention. Before telling the women's collective narrative in its collaged entirety, next I offer insight into my methods of data collection and analysis.

Researching Women's Stigmatized Voices

In 2005, noting the prevalence of the health condition and the underexamined and overhomogenized population of women attempting to navigate HPV identities and interventions, Ratzan warned that the HPV vaccine would require "ethical deliberation and societal choices" (p. 592). Specifically, Ratzan urged scholars to engage in "important dialogue to help set the course for the health of the next generation" (p. 592). Although mediated discussions largely delineated vaccination as an easy, widely accepted decision concerning every woman's health (see Horton, 2005), there was, and there continues to be, reason to believe that high-profile messages disseminated through public officials and media outlets may be working to reinforce stigma and thus complicate a woman's decision-making process. Specifically, advocates for HPV vaccination in the media and political spheres have been accused of homogenizing the voices, and thus the needs, of women with regards to HPV (Braun & Gavey, 1999). "Homogenization occurs through the suppression of individual voices and the acceptance of the omniscient voice of science as if it were our own" (Richardson, 2000, p. 925). In response to Ratzan's directive, and in the company of my own HPV-related experiences, I designed a study to explore the complex, sometimes contradictory, concerns of potential vaccine recipients.

Focus Group Interviews

For this study I conducted three focus group interviews with adult women ages 18 to 27 who were legally able to consider the vaccine when it was initially introduced to the market in June 2006. I selected this method of data collection on the basis of their resemblance to the feminist practice of consciousness raising as "focus groups can offer an in-depth understanding of perceptions, attitudes and beliefs about a particular topic, they can provide social and cultural interpretations of health-related topics, and they can generate unexpected or novel insights" (Lichtenstein, 2003, p. 2437). Each focus group consisted of three to six women. Although the "optimal size for a focus group is from 6 to 12 persons" (Lindlof & Taylor, 2011, p. 182), given the sensitive nature of this topic a more intimate atmosphere could be accomplished through a smaller gathering. In an attempt to help the participants "feel willing to express themselves on sensitive or long-repressed topics," this study aimed to produce a complementary interaction where participants broadly agreed on the view that the HPV vaccine was an important women's health issue but were then encouraged to add their own observations, experiences, and interpretations of that view (Lindlof & Taylor, p. 182).

Each focus group began with the viewing of textual materials—in the form of online Merck commercials,[1] a Merck brochure,[2] and a Merck magazine advertisement[3]—used to help orient the participants and provide a "push-off" to the discussion (Lindlof & Taylor, 2011, p. 183). As the researcher, I interjected a list of prepared questions and follow-up probes. Each focus group interview began with the open-ended question: "Can you please tell me what you know about HPV?" Each focus group interview lasted approximately 1 hour and 15 minutes and yielded over 75 pages of transcribed data. However, as recommended by Lindlof and Taylor, qualitative research should involve more than one type of data, and so I turned to personal interviews as a way to complement these general discussions by better illuminating specific concerns.

Individual Interviews

During one-on-one interviews, I sought to expand and clarify topics that were brought up during focus group interviews by asking each interview participant to explain, in as much detail as possible, their experiences with health practitioners, getting the vaccine, getting diagnosed with HPV, undergoing treatment for HPV, and engaging in dialogue with their partners about HPV. Because of an already established "shared frame of equality" and relationship with each of my participants, I engaged in a process of narrative interviewing, "the earliest known form of in-depth interviewing in the social sciences" (Lindlof & Taylor, p. 180; 181). Narrative interviews are the least structured type of interview because the goal is to find the most comfortable ground for each participant to tell his or her story.

I interviewed four women, and each personal interview ranged anywhere from one to three hours of dialogue and yielded an average of 26 pages of transcribed data. The interviews took place in public places, usually over a meal, and the conversation maintained a give-and-take quality that allowed each participant to bring up topics that they considered to be an important part of women's decisions about health. My selection of interview participants was guided by "purposeful sampling" (Lindlof & Taylor, 2011, p. 122) and each individual interviewee was a colleague and friend. During these semistructured, casual conversations concerns about the HPV vaccination were specified and illuminated.

Participant Observation

Over the course of four months, I tape recorded each focus group and narrative interview and took notes while the conversations unfolded. Each interview was followed by a recorded and written description of the location of each interview in order to help recount the event during the retelling of each woman's story. In addition to being an active member in each conversation, I visited the university health center twice and immersed myself in the information disseminated through these types of outlets. I also had three of my own gynecological appointments—one at a Planned Parenthood clinic to pick up birth control pills and another at a private office for my annual Pap smear appointment. The results of my Pap smear required a follow-up appointment. During each of these visits, I wrote about what I had been "*attracted to* and *convinced by*," and I wrote about what I read in pamphlets and official documents that I thought were "*meaningful*" in order to interpret what I read as a "meaningful *pattern*" (Goodall, 2000, p. 87). These methods of participant observation reveal the validity of the claim that "nothing that we know about a culture or about ourselves is free from *interpretation*" (Goodall, p. 87); for this reason, I also engaged in a process of introspection to recognize my own biases within the presentation of my data.

Introspection

In alignment with Sanger's (2003) concept of "polyvocality," this study intertwines the voices of the participants with my own voice as the researcher in order to expose the complicated nature of this women's health issue. To this end, and the fact that as a researcher I am unable to approach data without any assumptions (Lindlof & Taylor, 2011), I have incorporated personal accounts of my own experiences with HPV diagnosis, HPV treatment, and my own conversations regarding HPV vaccination. According to Sanger, "these pieces reveal intimate moments experienced by the [researcher] in an effort to give voice to the ways in which the process of consuming shapes the (feminist) self" (p. 36). Throughout this process, I too have become aware of my own social and cultural dilemmas associated with this health-related topic.

The following collective narrative lends insight into the complexities and constraints surrounding the HPV issue, in order to paint a more realistic view of the complications assumed with choosing to become vaccinated. Although the perceptions of the participants in these focus groups and interviews do not represent how all women's choices about HPV are restricted by current media depictions of this health issue, these results do offer a porthole into the concerns and opinions of the vaccine recipients. Ellingson (2008) reminds us that "scrutinizing the (mis)use of power and its accommodation or resistance is appropriate, even necessary to applied communication research that seeks to make a positive difference in the world" (p. 4). The view of the female vaccine recipient continues to be largely overlooked in mediated depictions of the health condition and the medical intervention. Contradictions, like the ones illuminated in this study, challenge the either/or nature of forced choices by problematizing the idea that "simple decisions are readily at hand" (Sowards & Renegar, 2004, p. 9).

The results of my thematic analysis of transcripts revealed that women communicated four factors as adding to their pressure to become vaccinated, and the subsequent limitation of choice: (1) generally, women are not well informed about health-related issues, (2) mediated depictions of health options advocate traditional gender-specific responsibilities, (3) women feel marginalized and disempowered by the STD discourse, and (4) women feel pressured to get the HPV vaccination. Although data was collected in the more specific, intimate, successive fashion described earlier, I present my findings here in a four-scene, collective narrative to illustrate the complexities of choice in women's conversations about HPV vaccination. The first scene, titled "Wait, how do you get HPV?" describes a general lack of information confronting women with regard to HPV. This lack of information is compounded by the dependence on media and healthcare providers to the neglect of personal effort. The second scene, titled "You deal with that, too," builds on the notion of media dependency and lends truth to the concern that media's depictions of women's responsibilities force them to be motivated by the needs of others instead of their own. This sentiment is often confounded when speaking about HPV because as the third scene, titled "It's like telling me you have breasts!" illustrates, HPV is often treated as a women's-only health issue. The final scene, titled "Does this mean I'm dirty?" relates to both media dependency and women's responsibilities regarding the concept of stigma as it relates to HPV. This last scene defines stigma as an ultimate silencer that is linked directly to each participant's inherent understanding of gendered responsibilities and the media depictions of the HPV problem, its cause, and its one solution.

"Wait, How Do You Get HPV?": Communicating Confusion

Us four ladies gathering around a coffee table, filling our glasses with wine, and chatting casually about cultural "rants and raves"; it's become a sort of tradition for us. My friends aren't necessarily diverse:

all white, all educated, all mid-twenties, all in relationships, but let me introduce them so we can best honor their subtleties:

Meet Bridget. I would describe her as affably rational. Bridget smiles when delivering criticism and worry and is currently admonishing belligerence by drinking water among the sea of winos.

Meet Sara. Sara is the type of woman I wish raised me. She comes across as level-headed, contributes opinions in the form of questions, and fools me into believing she would always have warm cookies for me to come home to.

Finally, meet Ashley. My friend Ashley makes me blush more than any person I know. Our annual meeting has just kicked off, I am two sips deep, and she has already used the word "cock" twice. Her RSVP email read as follows: "Can't wait to talk about the nether-region. Should we dress like our favorite STD?" Signed, "Seriously, Ashley."

"You know it's the pharmaceutical company paying for those commercials," Sara half questions, half states.

Ashley expresses worry with a twinge of anger: "How, how? Why?" Bridget adds, "They mark it up."

"Before they give it to you?!" Bridget continues, "She was gonna charge me 500 bucks so they were probably taking a really big cut of that."

Ashley holds her facial expression of disbelief mixed with agitation by letting her jaw fall partly open, and holding her head cocked to one side.

Sara shakes Ashley out of her visible disbelief by describing her last visit to the gynecologist: "I just had a gynecologist appointment and the lady was pretty much like 'OK, so now we should probably set up an appointment for you to get the vaccine' and I was like "um ... noooo, I don't really think I need it' and she was like 'well you know there is a cut-off and it is 26, so you gotta get moving on it,' and I was like 'well, I, um, I'm in a monogamous relationship, it's serious and I don't—' and she was just like 'this is a science issue, I don't understand why people are making it such a big deal. Just get it. It's smart.' I was like, 'OK, but no.' It was really tough for me to like hold my ground."

Bridget agrees and energetically moves to the edge of her seat on the couch, places her glass of water on the table, and brushes her hands together as if ridding them of crumbs. She stares at the table and through a smile that conveys perturbed disbelief with gynecological audacity interjects: "That was the exact same situation that I was in. I felt very strong-armed into it. I was like 'I need to talk to ... I'm gonna talk to my mom!"

We bounce the annoyed accounts of our troubles at the gynecologist back and forth.

Sara continues: "I was telling her, 'I already have HPV,' like, 'and I've had tons of different [treatments]' and then she's like, 'well that's just one strand you might not have the other one' and I was like, 'what? I don't understand.'"

Bridget adds: "they told me that it helps your body fight off the other strand. That was the rationale—apparently I had three so they're saying fight at least one of those. She said it can help fight, because there are like 50 strands."

I interject: "But that doesn't make sense, like biologically, because of how a vaccine works—you give yourself a small dose of it that your body can fight off, if you already have it, giving yourself a small dose of it isn't going to help your body fight it off more, right?"

This insight prompts a litany of technical questions about HPV and the vaccine, and as the moderator of the discussion I suddenly feel overwhelmed as if a cloud has opened over head and I am standing without an umbrella:

"Wait, how do you get HPV?"

"So are the four strands they know about—do all four of those lead to cervical cancer?"

"Girls who have low-risk strains, do they get warts?"

"But will you still test positive for HPV if you have [the non-cancer causing strains]?"

"Wait, can you test a guy for it?"

"If you have it or don't have it, can you get the vaccine and it's equally as effective?"

"Do you have to get your period to get the shot?"

"Do you have to be having sex to get [the vaccine]?"

"How much time between each shot?"

"You can just get [the shot] in your arm – nowhere weird right?"

"Is this a worldwide phenomenon?"

"Why is the age cut off 9–26?"

"So, can it go away?"

And then Sara interjects a comment that ceases the storm: "I keep telling all of these doctors that I know there are things going on with my cervix and like no one can get my records so they're just like starting over, but recently I just went to a new [gynecologist]and she's like 'alright, I don't think you'll want me cutting anything out but I'll look' and she's like looking and she's like 'there's no need for me to do this, just stick with me I think you've gotten like all sorts of miscommunication' and I was like: 'Thank you! Finally!' I don't know if this woman's right, but she certainly made me feel better because she didn't tell me I had to do something. Sometimes you trust that more, when they don't actually go and like cut you or do something like that just because they can, or just because they can make money. I just feel like sometimes that's being a better doctor by like holding back."

I ask, "What do you feel certain about HPV?" Sara hesitates in silence. We all stop chewing and wait for her reassuring remark.

"I feel certain that it's really important to get Pap smears. The only thing that is going to protect you is to get constantly monitored, and I think that that makes me feel more proactive about my health. But that's not advertised at all right now and that's really irritating."

* * *

Communication theory explains that media exposure affects individual judgments and behavior (McGuire, 1989). Research suggests that people, specifically women, are not well informed and cognitively active concerning social and political issues, and are therefore dependent on mediated messages to help them formulate decisions (Zaller, 1992; Kahneman & Tversky, 1984; Iyengar, 1991). This dependency results in women not being well informed about health issues and options due to (a) a narrow depiction of health issues disseminated through mediated campaigns, (b) a lack of information disseminated through healthcare providers, and (c) a lack of effort on the part of women to augment these limited understandings with alternative sources of information. Indeed, the media have been accused of keeping women "in a state of anxiety or punishment about their choices" (Baumgardner & Richards, 2000, p. 104). This exposes a potential consequence caused by an overreliance on media as a primary source of information used to make important decisions regarding health, especially if the information presented is confusing or incomplete. As was demonstrated, this concern was articulated across participant interviews, as mediated depictions of women's health issues have been linked to national health policy and funding priorities.

Ultimately, what these conversations reveal is that these women feel they have restricted choices regarding HPV vaccination, and that the connection between limited understanding of the health issue itself and its alternative solutions has much to do with a limited depiction of HPV across media. In media texts, discourse about women's issues often poses solutions to systematic problems as the need for women to take responsibility for their discontent by finding success within the system (Rockler, 2003). Communication scholars argue that the contemporary U.S. discourse is dominated by rhetoric that discourages citizens from contextualizing their personal problems within patriarchal power structures (Cloud, 1996, 1998; Peck, 1995; Rockler, 2003, 2006). They refer to this discourse as *therapeutic rhetoric* because of its ability to maintain the illusion that the overall system is fair (Jhally & Lewis, 1992: Rockler, 2003, p. 100). In order to keep from "repeating the paternalism of medicine that women's health activists have long fought against" (Braun & Gavey, 1999, p. 1471), however, women's empowerment concerning their sexual health is just as much about "learning how to do things for ourselves—including asking the rightquestions" as it is about "learning how not to do them on behalf of others" (Baumgardner & Richards, 2000, p. 30). As this scene demonstrates, with regard to women's health, sometimes this is easier said than done.

"You Will Deal with That Too": Communicating Responsibility

"You know what I think is funny? Remember last time we got together how I was saying that I didn't know if I should tell someone that I have HPV? Well, I am having sex right now."

I can't quite tell if Bridget pauses for the clap or only quiets in an attempt to politely receive the round of applause offered by us three women. She bashfully continues,

"So when I asked my gynecologists about it they were both like 'ooh not a big deal, a virus is a virus. Would you tell someone you had a cold?' You know?' So then when I was thinking about it; I had already been making-out with him and touching him when I started to ask them about it, you know what I mean? So I still haven't said anything. And I know he's gonna ask about the focus group tonight and I'm just gonna have to say, 'it's just about a subject.'" She laughs in a way that tells me she has never been any good at lying.

Sara attempts to relieve Bridget's concern and explains,

"I haven't told my boyfriend because ... don't know. I'm really torn because at this point it's been so long it's sort of shady. But at the same time it makes me feel like it's not relevant or important, and also it's like if guys aren't getting tested, then how do I know that he doesn't have it either. He's just gonna get upset about something that he may already have and doesn't know."

Ashley interjects, "It pisses me off that it is a woman's issue now. I mean, that really pisses me off. I mean, I don't know what to say. It puts all of the onus on women. I mean no other STD or ... But then it's like if you have to talk about sex than you are going to back yourself into a corner where [girls] will believe that sex is all [their] responsibility all the time."

Bridget responds with the jaded assumption: "But don't we anyways?"

Sara answers with a sing-song recollection of her daily sexual responsibilities: "You will take care of birth control. You will take care of the vaccination of HPV ..."

Bridget mocks: "If he does not want to put on a condom, you will tell him to put on the condom."

Ashley jumps in like she's been waiting on the sidelines in a game of double-dutch jump rope: "You will take care of the unexpected pregnancy—whatever way you take it—but you will deal with that too."

And suddenly it's as if the jump ropes clack to the ground in a deafening halt and we are each left holding on to an end of a rope, out of breath, in silence. We all look at each other and nod or smile only slightly, only enough to affirm that these duties somehow bond us together in a way that words can't describe.

* * *

When asked about HPV-related responsibilities, respondents in both the focus groups and personal interviews communicated a pressure to make the choice to get vaccinated on behalf of their partners. *Motivational displacement* is a term that refers to motivation that is derived from abandoning self-interests to meet the needs of others (Wood, 1994). According to Wood, motivational displacement occurs when "a person's motives for acting are centered on someone other than the self—the other takes prominence, and it is within the perspective of the other that a caregiver organizes her (or his) own goals, thoughts, and feelings" (p. 51). The consequence of motivational displacement is that it promotes "diminished autonomy" by reinforcing the belief that women are responsible to make decisions on account of other people's best interests and needs (Wood, 1994).

Gender-relational theory indicates that women are designated as "the traditional guardians of health" (Lichtenstein, 2004, p. 371). Not only are women expected to act in their own best health-related interest, they are also expected to be the custodians of health for men, children, and families (Miles, 1991; Sabo, 2000). This places certain pressures on women making choices concerning their own sexual health. These dominant values are reinforced in women's stories of their interactions with healthcare providers, and their motivation for considering vaccination on account of the health and well-being of their current partners and future children. Responsibility requires women to experience another person's needs as their own, so much so that these women expressed the risk of beginning to make choices about their own health in terms of another person's needs.

"It's Like Telling Me You Have Breasts!": Communicating Sex

After refilling her water, on her return from the kitchen Bridget begins, "You know, [the vaccine is] kinda, like, putting extra pressure on a different generation of people—it's like it's a new problem for our generation and those after us, and it's not something that those people who make the drugs and make the policies are ever gonna have to think about for themselves."

Over the course of these focus groups, almost every one of the women makes reference to the previous generation's opinion about

HPV. *Although each of us has been dutifully kicked out of the nest, these new commercials have prompted concerned maternal phone calls from far and wide.*

"My mom was like 'you need to get this shot' and I was like, 'well, why? I'm not gonna have sex with anyone besides X for the rest of my life' and she was like, 'oh well you should get it' and I felt like it was impeding on my relationship and that like if you don't get [the shot] then you're gonna be sorry like their leading you to not trust [your boyfriend]. I mean granted, I don't live in denial, I know shit happens. ..."

Sara offers up a counter-approach: "I mean you could turn it around on your mom, not that she has a choice, but she's not vaccinated — she's doing okay, knock on wood."

Bridget includes her mother's voice in a way that makes me want to meet her and wish she was the one who gave me my sex-talk: "Every woman gets HPV, Bridget, I do not know a woman who does not have HPV. It's like telling them you have breasts!" *Bridget reassumes her articulate, calm demeanor and clarifies:* "For [that generation] it's like chicken pox or like the flu, it's something every woman gets, and you get it taken care of, and that's it, and for us it's become this whole like 'should I tell about the STD that I have contracted?'"

Sara vents, "It just seems like this whole HPV thing is wrought with contradiction where it's like, 'Oh it's just a virus, everyone has it. Oh talk about it,' but then everyone is worried that people are going to go out and have sex like crazy!"

"And THIS is why no one in the media wants to talk about HPV like it's an STD," *Bridget quips.*

"Everyone that is in the media is talking about [HPV] like cancer. No one wants to talk about it like it's a sexually transmitted disease OR that it's a virus." *Sara explains in a reassuring, there's-nothing-we-can-do-about-it tone. She continues,* "It's cuz you can't sell a vaccine that's like, 'Here's a virus that there is a 3% chance of getting cancer from.' You can't do that. And I think that that is why it has been reframed like that, right?"

I nod, agreeing.

"But, I feel like it would have more of an impact if it was framed like an STD, not cancer," *interjects Ashley.* "I feel like 12- to 20-year-olds are more concerned with getting an STD than cancer. Because they're still invincible, so of course they're not going to get cancer. But getting an STD is right on their minds because sex is on their minds. So if the media explained [HPV] like 'Yo, this is an STD and it's not adorable' then [people] might take it more to heart because they think: 'I'm never gonna get cancer.'"

Bridget wonders, "I don't know because when people hear STD they think dirty, sick. I don't think they think they are going to die."

Sara adds, while nodding, "And you also hear the word cancer and think of the word victim and if you hear the word STD you think of like 'slut.'"

"It's interesting that you just said the word slut because that's like totally 'girl,'" confesses Bridget.

"Yeah, I mean, I don't like that word at all, but it's like exactly what I think of," confesses Sara as well.

"Yeah, the word that popped into my head was definitely not 'man-whore,' laughs Bridget.

Sara continues to defend her case, "If you say cancer you think victim ... you think patient. But when you say STD you don't think of patients; you think more of like people who deserve it. And I know that is totally bad to think, especially from a person who has had a long past with HPV, but I totally think that."

I jump in with a cathartic confession and explain that "when I was diagnosed I felt like I deserved it. I almost embodied that idea."

Instead of consonance, Bridget offers her similar experience: "The reason I can't talk to my boyfriend about it is because I feel dirty."

Sara validates Bridget's concern by interjecting that she has had a guy break up with her because she told him that she had HPV: "And his mom is a nurse!" she adds for a more dramatic effect. "After I had that reaction, I have been more hesitant to tell people."

Leave it to Ashley to put Sara on the spot, "Does your current boyfriend know?"

Sara hesitates, breaks eye contact with all of us, then confidently states, "I have had enough people tell me that it is okay that I don't say anything. Sometimes that's what you need. Have you ever heard of the difference between secrecy and privacy? Secrecy is actually keeping something from someone that directly affects them, whereas privacy is just keeping something to yourself. So it depends on how you look at HPV. If you are looking at it like a virus, then it would have to do with privacy, but if you are looking at it like an STD that could possibly kill then that would be secrecy. But I am trying to look at it more like a virus—so maybe that's my justification. And then it's like, if this is someone you are going to stay with forever and they're not going to get cervical cancer, then why tell them? Why does it matter to them? I understand that if you're casually dating, you can give it to your next love of your life."

"... That's what I'm thinking—that they would give it to the next girl," Ashley worries. "That's the girl I am thinking about."

* * *

Within these focus groups, how women talk about diagnosis and disclosure of their HPV status revealed worries surrounding a perpetual stigma propagated by the belief that testing positive for an STD connotes unfaith-fulness and/or irresponsible behavior. When asked about the role of the media in regard to HPV-related stigma, responses suggested that hiding the sexual nature of the disease throughout the public sphere works to validate HPV's link to promiscuity as a "women's only" problem. This finding corresponds with Braun and Gavey's (1999) conviction that "the suppression of sexual risk factor information actually [strengthens] its status as stigma-invoking information" (p. 1473). Across disciplines, most research concerning STDs and stigma tends to focus on how stigma affects a person's decision to get tested (Barth, Cook, Downs, Switzer, & Fischoff, 2002; Fortenberry et al., 2002; Lichtenstein, 2003, 2004; Lindemann, 1988). Most studies conclude that stigma and shame associated with a possible positive STD status deter people from getting tested, especially for diseases without a cure like AIDS/ HIV (Lichtenstein, 2003). Because of the relatively new buzz surrounding HPV, current studies have not explored how stigma and shame may affect a person's decision to become vaccinated—a preventative measure as opposed to the less agentic measure of testing positive for an incurable disease and "telling someone" about that status.

Despite the fact that both men and women carry HPV and are jointly responsible for this "hidden epidemic," HPV has been largely designated a women's health issue (Colgrove, 2006, p. 2390). More specifically, as this last scene demonstrated, for women considering the vaccination HPV feels like *this* generation's women's health issue. This can be attributed to a number of reasons: Mediated depictions have emphasized cervical can-cer as the worst case scenario for an HPV diagnosis despite its fatal link to other forms of head, neck, and anal cancer, and, up until 2009, only females were approved to get vaccinated. Johnson and Hoffman (1994) explained that women's medical problems are often described by the media and understood as deviations from the norm, and Ruzek, Olesen, and Clarke (1997) suggest that this is because the media takes women's health issues out of context and reports unrealistic views of cures and progress. For these reasons, and as this last scene illustrates, discussion about GARDASIL® and HPV has been shaped by mediated assumptions about girls' and women's lives rather than by biological concerns (Horton, 2005; Kessler & Wood, 2007). In sum, links to deviant behavior and unrealistic understandings of HPV's causes and cures have perpetuated an image of the disease that designates it as a women's-only health issue and one with stigmatizing consequences for the next generation of sexually active females.

"Does this Mean I'm Dirty?": Communicating Stigma

Bridget ends our evening together with a flippantly serious statistic: "Did you know that 96% of us have it and now 96% of us are dirty.

And, we have to find out if we have it—so it's that responsibility as well. We have to tell people."

Sara mocks a healthcare professional by sitting up straight, pretending to peer over a pair of glasses, and shaking her head from side to side as she scolds each of us: *"96% of you have to tell your boyfriends or potential dates."*

Ashley has managed to dodge the scolding glance by maintaining eye contact with the bowl of frosted animal cookies and only looks up to boldly ask: *"Wait, what's your current status?"*

I admire her defiant ability to ask what's on her mind despite social privacy boundaries. Her mouth full of cookies delivers the uncomfortable question with an air of childish curiosity, and Bridget responds.

"I think they said—I don't even know how many strains I had—that's the thing, I had abnormal cells on my cervix, they didn't test for HPV they just thought it was HPV."

Sara interjects: *"I went in for an annual Pap smear and they tested [me] and they were like 'Ooh you have abnormal cells,' and then they tested for HPV, and I don't even remember at this point but it must have come back and must have been something similar to that? Afterwards, I had to go for every six months for like two years and then I was like 'clean' for two years."*

Ashley continues her line of prying: *"Sara, did you tell your boyfriend?"*

Sara doesn't hesitate: *"If I've had two years of clean Pap smears, then it makes me feel like it's not relevant or important, right?"*

And so, annually ladies across America hold their breath for clean bills of health, hoping and wishing to be part of the chosen few; to come out on top and avoid awkward disclosures. Today I received my *"bill of health."*

Dear Ms. Malkowski,

Your Pap smear revealed changes called ASC-US or atypical squamous cells of undetermined significance. This is felt to be a mild abnormality and usually resolves on its own. It is often due to the human papilloma virus or HPV. ... It is our policy to perform this testing for "high-risk" strains of HPV in patients with ASC-US. These high-risk strains may predispose a patient to develop a more severe cervical disorder. Your test indicated that there is NO EVIDENCE of high-risk HPV strains. Therefore, our recommendation is that you simply repeat your Pap smear in one year.

Sincerely,

Student Health Services

I have translated this professional correspondence in order to best convey the undertones prevalent only to those women who understand the significance of their odds:

Dear Jennifer,
Congratulations! You have been selected from an over-qualified pool of applicants as achieving this year's HPV-Negative Honorable Status. This award designates you as part of the top 4% of the female population and we encourage you to disclose this status to past, present, and future intimate-others as both a testament to faithfulness and sexual responsibility. We are a proud sponsor of this annual event as we fervently believe the prospect of receiving this prestigious status will work to motivate women in both conduct and attitude. Thank you for your participation and we look forward to your application next year!
Sincerely,
Center for Disease Control and Prevention

* * *

Ultimately, the findings from this study reveal a tendency for women to feel like they have restricted choices regarding HPV vaccination. Most scholars agree that it is time to increase awareness of the preventability of STDs and, furthermore, promote sex education and health-promoting messages as ways to destigmatize the overall situation (Lichtenstein, 2004). However, "as we move toward more public awareness of women's health issues in the next 10 years it is imperative that the media provide a comprehensive look at issues that affect their audiences—and there is no better institution to provide this scrutiny than the media, as they pursue the public service function of providing women and the general population with necessary information to make informed decisions" (Andsager & Powers, 2001, p. 182). The connections between women's limited understanding of the health issue itself and alternative options has much to do with a limited depiction of HPV across media outlets.

The ethical principle of women's rights to make informed choices has helped women learn to do their research in order to ask tough questions and demand that doctors take their ailments seriously (Braun & Gavey; Rosen). Because of this impulse and opportunity, according to third-wave feminism, "all women have the power to choose a successful and fulfilling path and must take personal responsibility for doing so" (Rockler, 2006, p. 251). However, Bunkle (1990) noted that the very notion of health-related choices is problematic because it often ignores other variables that impact an individual's ability to make health choices. Results from this study illuminated a dependency on mediated depictions of HPV that worked to complicate women's "power to choose." Indeed, findings from this study suggest that women remain largely underinformed, underaddressed, and yet overly exposed to mediated depictions of HPV.

Findings from this study articulate the need for public health officials and media outlets to communicate a more honest depiction of the disease, its causes, and the many different preventative options available to both sexually active women *and* men. Although this particular group of participants could be described as homogeneous, demographically speaking, even within this group of similar others complications, contradictions, and disagreements arose concerning the best course of action in relation to HPV. Future research should seek to diversify the participant pool as to consider a more diverse collection of women's narratives concerning HPV. That being said, much more might still be gained by further investigating how seemingly homogeneous groups of women experience intragroup divides and differences that impede each woman's ability to evaluate personal needs and act accordingly. Identifying the mechanisms of difference within certain health populations may, in turn, help women to navigate health contexts more generally.

I have identified three factors contributing to women's decisions about health-related practices that reveal laden contradictions regarding HPV options. Specifically, women are not informed, but they feel responsible for making informed decisions, and women feel disempowered and marginalized by this topic but are expected to lead its solution. To illustrate these juxtapositions, recall Ashley's concern, "I know very little. I know what's on the commercials, and I know that there is a vaccine for it and I think that you need to get three shots. I don't know why there are three, I don't know why you have to get them, and I don't know who can get that," paired against the health practitioner's statement, "so, will you be getting the HPV vaccine?" followed by her coax that "It's just the responsible, healthy decision." Furthermore, an understanding of HPV as an STD instigated conversation surrounding the burden of women's stigmatized sexuality.

Also recall that Sara explained that "[i]f you hear the word STD you think of like 'slut'," and Bridget diagnosed that this definition mixed with the prevalence of HPV meant that "96% of [women] are dirty." Yet, despite these stigmatizing factors, Sara reminded us that the mediated messages that define HPV—namely, the "Tell Someone" campaign—communicates that "96% of [women] have to tell your boyfriends or potential dates" that they have tested positive for HPV. By framing the HPV vaccine as cancer prevention, the media implicitly validate the stigma associated with STDs whose consequences fall disproportionately on women. This stigma works to silence opinions about the vaccine and demands for alternative options, providing women with a false dichotomy: You can either get the vaccine to protect yourself and those you love, or you can choose not to protect yourself against cancer. According to Sowards and Renegar (2004), "The polarizations and forced choices of the status quo often create situations where it is impossible to enact authentic, self-created decisions" (p. 13). This dichotomy becomes significant in recognizing the potential consequences assumed when women act out of necessity rather than choice.

In the media, the HPV epidemic has been simplified to reflect one option as the only "responsible" choice. By framing the HPV vaccine as a "choice," Merck's campaign ignores the fact that protection from STDs and cervical cancer requires more than just a vaccine. Framing HPV protection as a "choice" may work to perpetuate the gendered stigma associated with STDs by implicitly suggesting that girls who choose to be sexually active, and who choose to not get the vaccine, are choosing to get HPV. By framing cervical cancer protection as a "choice," this media campaign runs the risk of creating a situation where women who can't get vaccinated or who "choose" not to get vaccinated and contract cervical cancer years from now may be blamed for their condition. "Such concerns about victim-blaming are particularly pertinent in this area, given that there are no straightforward behavioural [sic] choices that can be recommended to guarantee absolute protection from the sexual transmission of HPV" (Braun & Gavey, 1999, p. 1472). The potentially stigmatizing consequences of downplaying this understanding of the nature of HPV and the limited protection that the vaccine can offer poses the risk of lending false hope to women who decide to get the vaccine and placing stigma and blame on the shoulders of future cervical cancer victims.

Although information about sexuality, STDs, and cervical cancer proved to be the central accomplishment of the women's health movement (see Horton, 2005), research continues to find that women have little or no knowledge about the risk factors for cervical cancer. And results from this study demonstrate the ways that a lack of knowledge contributes to isolated, confusing experiences of HPV diagnosis, treatment, and prevention. The media have been targeted as a "major source of medical information" that can be "particularly important in educating policymakers and the general public about new scientific advances" (Calloway et al., 2006, p. 808; Hornik, 1997) like the HPV vaccine. However, given its persuasive potential, researchers have warned that "effective HPV education must include information about transmission, prevention, treatment, and cervical carcinoma risk ... and provide a balance between accurate discussion of cancer risk and reassurance that following recommended screening practices will reduce risk to negligible levels" (Anhang, Wright, Smock, & Goldie, 2003, p. 315, as to avoid inciting unnecessary senses of urgency and anxiety concerning the health condition (Braun & Gavey). Although the three-scene narrative presented in these pages was rendered only from the stories and insights of a few women, we see that complexities, confusion, and contradictions, and thus urgency and anxiety, necessarily abound. The three themes identified here offer an initial means by which women can begin to understand their complicated experiences with HPV as part of a larger shared reality, one characterized by urgency and anxiety but one that is ultimately navigable as well.

Notes

1. Choose to be one less. (2007). *Merck* [Commercial]. Retrieved April, 4, 2008, from http://www.gardasil.com/tv-commercial-for-gardasil.html; Tell someone. (2006). *Merck* [Commercial]. Retrieved April, 4, 2008, from http://hpv.com/hpv-resources.html?WT.srch=1&WT.mc_id=GR042.
2. Tell Someone [Brochure]. (2006). Merck: USA.
3. Learn the truth about HPV [Advertisement]. (2007, December). *Glamour*, 219–224.

References

Andsager, J. L., & Powers, A. (2001). Framing women's health with a sense-making approach: Magazine coverage of breast cancer and implants. *Health Communication, 13*, 163–185.

Anhang, R., Wright, T. C., Smock, L., & Goldie, S. J. (2003). Women's desired information about human papillomavirus. *Cancer, 100*, 315–320.

Barth, K. R., Cook, R. L. Downs, J. S., Switzer, G. E., & Fischhoff, B. (2002). Social stigma and negative consequences: Factors that influence college students' decisions to seek testing for sexually transmitted infections. *Journal of American College Health, 50*, 153–159.

Baumgardner, J., & Richards, A. (2000). *Manifesta: Young women, feminism, and the future.* New York: Farrar, Straus & Giroux.

Bickley, J. (1987). Safety screen or smoke screen? *New Zealand Nursing Journal, 81*, 10–12.

Braun, V., & Gavey, N. (1999). "With the best of reasons": Cervical cancer prevention policy and the suppression of sexual risk factor information. *Social Science and Medicine, 48*,1463–1474.

Bunkle, P. (1990). Women and power: How can we change the system. *Fourth International Congress of Women's Health Issues.* Massey University, Palmerston North, New Zealand Papers.

Calloway, C., Jorgensen, C. M., Saraiya, M., & Tsui, J. (2006). A content analysis of news coverage of the HPV vaccine by U.S. newspapers, January 2002–June 2005. *Journal of Women's Health, 15*, 803–809.

Campbell, K. K. (2005). The rhetoric of women's liberation: An oxymoron. *Quarterly Journal of Speech, 59*, 74–86.

Centers for Disease Control and Prevention. (2006, August). *HPV vaccine questions and answers.* Retrieved February 22, 2007, from http://www.cdc.gov/std/hpv/STDFact-HPV-vaccine.htm.

Cloud, D. L. (1996). Hegemony or concordance? The rhetoric of tokenism in "Oprah" Winfrey's rags-to-riches biography. *Critical Studies in Mass Communication, 13*, 115–137.

Cloud, D. L. (1998). *Control and consolation in American culture and politics: Rhetoric of therapy.* Thousand Oaks, CA: Sage.

Colgrove, J. (2006). The ethics of politics of compulsory HPV vaccination. *New England Journal of Medicine, 354*, 2645–2654.

Dederer, C. (2007, February 18). Pitching protection to both mothers and daughters. *New York Times.* Retrieved March 16, 2007, from http://www.newyorktimes.com.

Dow, B. J. (1996). *Prime-time feminism: Television, media culture, and the women's movement since 1970.* Philadelphia: University of Pennsylvania Press.

Ellingson, L. L. (2008). Ethnography in applied communication research. In L. R. Frey & K. Cissna (Eds.), *The handbook of applied communication research.* Mahwah, NJ: Erlbaum.

Fortenberry, J. D., McFarlane, M., Bleakley, A., Bull, S., Fishbein, M., Grimley, D. M., et al. (2002). Relationships of stigma and shame to gonorrhea and HIV screening. *American Journal of Public Health, 92,* 378–381.

Goodall, H. L. (2000). *Writing the new ethnography.* Walnut Creek, CA: Altamira Press.

Hornik, R. (1997). Public health education and communication as policy instruments for bringing about change in behavior. In M. E. Goldberg, M. Fishbein, & S. E. Middlestadt (Eds.), *Social marketing: Theoretical and practical perspectives.* Mahwah, NJ: Erlbaum.

Horton, M. J. (2005). A shot against cervical cancer: A stunning new youth vaccine promises to prevent the deadly disease—but will parents go for it? *Ms. Magazine.* Retrieved September 28, 2007, from http://www.msmagazine.com/summer2005/cervicalcancer.asp.

Iyengar, S. (1991). *Is anyone responsible?* Chicago: University of Chicago Press.

Jhally, S., & Lewis, J. (1992). *Enlightened racism: The Cosby Show, audiences, and the myth of the American dream.* Boulder, CO: Westview.

Johnson, K., & Hoffman, E. (1994). Women's health and curriculum transformation: The role of medical specialization. In A. J. Dan (Ed.), *Refreshing women's health* (pp. 27–39). Thousand Oaks, CA: Sage.

Kahn, J. A., Slap, G. B., Bernstein, D. I., Kollar, L. M., Tissot, A. M., Hillard, P. A., et al. (2005). Psychological, behavioral, and interpersonal impact of human papillomavirus and Pap test results. *Journal of Women's Health, 14,* 650–659.

Kahneman, D., & Tversky, A. (1984). Choice, values, and frames. *Political Communication, 10,* 55–76.

Kessler, B., & Wood, S. (2007). A shot in the dark: What-and who- is behind the marketing of *GARDASIL®? Ms. Magazine, 36,* 27–28, 32.

Lichtenstein, B. (2003). Stigma as a barrier to treatment of sexually transmitted infection in the American Deep South: Issues of race, gender and poverty. *Social Science and Medicine, 57,* 2435–2445.

Lichtenstein, B. (2004). Caught at the clinic: African American men, stigma, and STI treatement in the Deep South. *Gender and Society, 18,* 369–388.

Lindemann, C. (1988). Counseling issues in disclosure of sexually transmitted disease. In M. Rodway & M. Wright (Eds.), *Decade of the plague: The sociopsychological ramifications of STD* (pp. 59–69). New York: Harrington Park Press.

Lindlof, T., & Taylor, B. (2011). *Qualitative communication research methods* (3rd ed.). Thousand Oaks, CA: Sage.

McGuire, W. J. (1989). Theoretical foundations of campaigns. In R. E. Rice & C. K. Atkin (Eds.), *Public communication campaigns* (2nd ed., pp. 43–65). Newbury Park, CA: Sage.

Merck launches national advertising campaign for *GARDASIL®*, Merck's new cervical cancer vaccine. (November 23, 2006). *Medical News Today.* Retrieved September 9, 2008, from www.medicalnewstoday.com.

Miles, A. (1991). *Women, health and medicine.* Buckingham, UK: Open University Press.

Peck, J. (1995). TV talk shows as therapeutic discourse: The ideological labor of the televised talking cure. *Communication Theory, 5,* 58–81.

Ratzan, S. C. (2005). Advancing an agenda on risk and chronic disease [Editorial]. *Journal of Health Communication, 10,* 591–592.

Richardson, L. (2000). Writing: A method of inquiry. In N. Denzin & Y. Lincoln (Eds.), *Handbook of qualitative research* (2nd ed.) (pp. 923–948). Thousand Oaks, CA: Sage.

Rockler, N. R. (2003). Entertainment, the personal, and the political: Therapeutic rhetoric and popular culture controversies. *Communication Review, 6,* 97–115.

Rockler, N. R. (2006). "Be your own windkeeper": Friends, feminism, and rhetorical strategies of depoliticization. *Women's Studies in Communication, 29,* 244–264.

Rosen, R. (2000). *The world split open: How the modern women's movement changed America.* New York: Penguin Books.

Ruzek, S. B. (1978). *The women's health movement: Feminist alternatives to medical control.* New York: Praeger.

Ruzek, S. B., Olesen, V. L., & Clarke, A. E. (1997). *Women's health: Complexities and differences.* Columbus: Ohio State University Press.

Sabo, D. (2000). Men's health studies: Origins and trends. *Journal of American College Health, 49,* 133–142.

Sanger, P. C. (2003). Living and writing feminist ethnographies: Threads in a quilt stitched from the heart. In R. P. Clair (Ed.), *Expressions of ethnography: Novel approaches to qualitative methods.* Albany: State University of New York Press.

Sowards, S. K., & Renegar, V. R. (2004). The rhetorical functions of consciousness-raising in third wave feminism. *Communication Studies, 55,* 535–552.

Wood, J. T. (1994). *Who cares?: Women, care, and culture.* Carbondale: Southern Illinois University Press.

Zaller, J. R. (1992). *The nature and origins of mass opinion.* New York: Cambridge University Press.

11 American Menstruation Rhetoric as Sanitized Discourse
Iterating Stigma through Print Advertisements

Erika M. Thomas

Introduction

Whether it is referred to as the "the curse," "my red-headed friend," or "that time of the month," the prominent use of euphemisms in American culture suggests that menstruation has been treated more as a disorder or a dirty secret than as a natural element of the female reproductive cycle.[1] In contrast, doctors and biologists describe menstruation as a straightforward process: From the onset of puberty, the uterine wall builds up and in the absence of fertilization sheds a nutrient and blood-filled lining. This scientific perspective of menstruation as an essential element of human reproduction represents a significant shift from the classical origins of understanding menstruation in various cultures, but nonetheless, menstruation remains a taboo topic, dating back to ancient times. Despite progressive social relations and education, American discourses depict menstruation as an act that is threatening and socially harmful to women, which in turn creates implications for the health and well-being of women.

This chapter argues that the stigmatized communication surrounding menstruation is closely linked to the discourse of repression and has become an accepted ideology in American consumer culture. My analysis uses Foucault's theory of the repressive hypothesis to demonstrate how modern "talk" surrounding feminine hygiene products involves particular discursive strategies to create shame around the issues of women's bodies and to sell products. I contend that print advertisements in women's magazines play upon the fears and hopes of menstruating women, revealing how the modern taboo shapes public discourse about menstruation. Women thereby experience menstruation in a particular way, reinforcing the taboo for capitalist gain and risking their health to maintain cultural expectations. Although the rhetorical trend examined is one that is perpetuated by the marketing and consumer media, it directly impacts women's healthcare and stigmatizes women's bodies. Thus, this chapter exposes the stigmatized messages surrounding menstruation in order to recognize a potential barrier that stonewalls dialogues about women's reproductive health and silences women's voices on the subject.

The Menstruation Taboo

Western culture has long treated menstruation as threatening or dirty. Medical writings and dominant metaphors about menstruation have historically negative connotations that maintain stigmas and reinforce patriarchy (Martin, 1987). Ancient Greece is one early society that constructed differences between genders on the premise of a hierarchy of fluid, which resulted in the subordination of women.

> For Aristotle, therefore, and for the long tradition founded in his thought, the generative substances are interconvertible elements in the economy of a single-sex body whose higher form is male. As physiological fluids they are not distinctive and different in kind, but the lighter shades of biological chiaroscuro drawn in blood.
>
> (Laqueur, 1990, p. 42)

Examining the menstruation taboo reveals a number of trends. Historically, the menstruation was viewed as a larger threat to society because menstruating women were viewed as dangerous to others. In particular, a menstruating woman's offspring, husband, family, and even other men in her community were believed to be at risk of curses, diseases, and even death. The biblical book of Leviticus referenced women's impure effects on others (Bullough & Bullough, 1995, p. 107), and women were often confined in spaces during their menses because of the various dangers it was believed they posed to society. It was commonly believed that intercourse with a menstruating woman would cause harm to men (Crawford, 1981, p. 61) or that a monstrous or deformed child would be born to any woman who conceived while she was menstruating (Niccoli, 1990, p. 8). Such radical beliefs continued in the nineteenth century, when A.F.A. King, a physician writing during 1875, argued that intercourse during menses resulted in gonorrhea (Bullough & Bullough, p. 112), and other medical texts claimed that men would thereby acquire leprosy (Niccoli, p. 10). These examples illustrate that, in earlier centuries, menstruating women were viewed as more of a danger to others than to themselves.

Despite Western culture's dissipation of this logic, the menstrual taboo is ever present in the West. However, transgressing the code now jeopardizes a different target. Rather than primarily threatening those around them with pollution, *women themselves* are threatened by the danger of embarrassment, ostracism, or dirt caused by their own menstruation. Rierdan and Hastings (1990) explain that the "medicalizing of menstruation has resulted from even well-informed educators" and that "openness" about the subject continues to "perpetuate the bias of viewing menstruation as essentially a matter of hygiene and disease" (p. 20). Many women claim they feel "dirty" or "disgusting" when menstruating. Martin (1987) states that the taboo is consistently discussed in her interviews with women representing diverse classes and ethnic identities. She explains, "Because most women are aware that in our general cultural view menstruation is dirty, they are still stuck with the 'hassle': most centrally no one must ever see you dealing with the mechanics of keeping up with the disgusting mess, and you must never fail to keep the disgusting mess from showing on your clothes, furniture or the floor" (Martin, 1987, p. 93). Furthermore, society's vocabulary keeps women feeling self-conscious about menstruating. Lee and Sasser-Coen (1996) identify common words and jargon that imply or describe female genitalia as "smelly" and "unpleasant." Because gendered identities are intricately linked to bodies, menstruating girls and women are internally oppressed and experience embarrassment and shame. Interviews with women revealed fears of "showing evidence of wearing pads or stain-ing garments and sheets" and the pressure to "conceal and hide evidence of menstruation" (p. 81). Lee and Sasser-Coen conclude: "language and forms of knowledge about the female body uphold practices and justify ideas, behaviors, and policies that maintain patriarchal social relations and func-tion symbolically to represent understandings of women's roles" (p. 72).

Making women themselves the ones threatened by menstruation pri-vatizes their bodily issues and leads to women condoning the shift to take responsibility for control of their "leaky" bodies. According to Crawford (1981), women in most Western countries wanted the issue to remain a private topic. Negative feelings stemming from the taboo and pressure for secrecy and silence surrounding the topic of menstruation reinforce women's feelings of fear and embarrassment and the need to privatize their natural cycle. According to Rierdan and Hastings (1990), even women writ-ers who broach the subject of menstruation are restrained. Rierdan and Hastings (1990) argue that although psychological research on menstruation in women's lives has been done, the studies are often inaccessible and imper-sonal (Rierdan & Hastings, pp. 23–24). Additionally, Martin highlights the problems with present scientific writings and shows how menstruation, seen as a failed production, leads to our negative view of the process (Martin, p. 48). Even if not all texts contain negative terminology in the description of menstruation, scientific writings reflect the unconscious attitudes of a culture. These examples provide evidence that a modern menstruation taboo has emerged in the 20th century. Although it may seem tolerable and almost acceptable in comparison to the early taboos and practices followed by early cultures, disciplinary practices and etiquette that safeguard menstrual blood and reinforce the belief that menstruation is something to be controlled, concealed, and rejected reproduce gender differences that discriminate against women.

Understanding Menstruation through the Repressive Hypothesis

The characteristics surrounding the rhetoric of menstruation emulate the discursive trends of sexually repressed populations. Michel Foucault's gene-alogy, *The History of Sexuality* (1978), traces the repressive hypothesis theory, which contributes to understanding the historical narrative of the 21st-century discourse surrounding menstruation politics.

Foucault (1978) explains that in the 17th century explicit sexual discourses in the public sphere were deemed inappropriate by the Victorian bourgeoisie. Foucault (1978) states, "Sexuality was carefully confined; it moved into the home. The conjugal family took custody of it and absorbed it into the serious function of reproduction. On the subject of sex, silence became the rule" (p. 3). As a result of Puritanism's "triple edict of taboo, nonexistence and silence," the discussion of sexual conduct was censored from public discourse; it was only permitted within the sanctity of the marriage, church confessionals, mental institutions, and brothels (Foucault, 1978, pp. 4–5).

Although the strict limitations placed on sexual discourse appeared to eradicate most public talk of sex, Foucault's examination reveals an explosion of authorized discourses in certain spaces. In short, the restriction of sexuality to the private sphere did not "succeed" in the Victorian era. Instead, this repression required a new type of sexual rhetoric; extensive discourse about sexuality in various coded forms pervaded the public. He states: "But this was not a plain and simple imposition of silence. Rather, it was a new regime of discourses. Not any less was said about it; on the contrary. But things were said in a different way; it was different people who said them, from different points of view, and in order to obtain different results" (Foucault, 1978, p. 27). Despite the intense regulations, the early 18th century witnessed the creation of multiple discourses that discussed sex while simultaneously regulating and masking it. The more society attempted to control and repress sexual discourse, the more attention sex proliferated throughout society. Foucault explains this phenomenon as the "repressive hypothesis."

> At their level of discourses and their domains, however, practically the opposite phenomenon occurred. There was a steady proliferation of discourses concerned with sex—specific discourses different from one another both by their form and by their object: a discursive ferment that gathered momentum from the eighteenth century onward.
>
> (Foucault, 1978, p. 18)

The emerging discourses were highly coded and characterized by new "rules," such as insinuation and symbolism. Foucault (1978) explains:

> A whole rhetoric of allusion and metaphor was codified. Without question, new rules of propriety screened out some words: there was a policing of statements. A control over enunciations as well: where and when it was not possible to talk about such things became much more strictly defined; in which circumstances, among which speakers and within which social relationships. (p. 17–18)

Sexuality was not completely hidden or removed from public discourse; its presence was unavoidable. Construction of new discursive approaches allowed discussion of sexuality publicly while simultaneously maintaining it as a "private matter." Sustaining this unstable arrangement required a public vigilance that encouraged and demanded discourse. This authorized discourse dictated the ways in which citizens were to manage, discuss, and enact their sexuality. Foucault illustrates that discourse was one way to enact biopower over populations and the sexuality and bodies of individuals living in the 19th century.

Although our contemporary medical community has alleviated much of this initial medical pathology surrounding sexuality and women's bodies, additional and severe "agencies of control" have emerged and remain present in contemporary American society. Despite the apparent proliferation of sexual discourses, explicit issues of reproduction remain confined to the private sphere. Current advertisements illustrate that, despite the limits on sexual discourse, a secretive, yet obsessive, discourse around menstruation remains present. Advertisements attempting to sell feminine hygiene products are present on television and in magazines, yet licit and shameless discourse is rarely used. Instead, censorship, symbolism, and euphemisms are used to safely cover up the inappropriate and dangerous discourse. This pattern has clearly been seen since the 1920s when menstrual products first appeared in advertising. Today, society still regulates the threat. Lee and Sasser-Coen (1996) explain: "Society maintains taboos against positive discussions of menarche and menstruation, and, as a result, reinforces cultural values that see menstrual blood as dirty and smelly, polluting, and contaminating" (pp. 68–69).

Because menstruation remains a censored topic in the private sphere, alternative discourses have emerged within advertising campaigns to reinforce menstruation as private and taboo. As Foucault's theory illustrates, repression of discourse and confinement to the private sphere cannot succeed. When repression occurs, attempting to conceal voices on the subject, a proliferation of coded, public discourse develops and this, in turn, further draws attention to it. Thus, repression backfires and results in often newly invented, coded discourses that emerge in the public sphere.

The Repressive Hypothesis in the Contemporary Menstruation Taboo

Historical accounts of society's attitudes toward menstruation reveal that discourse about menses was largely relegated to the private sphere prior to the 20th century. As with discourse surrounding sexuality, Victorian society viewed public discussions about menstruation and women's personal hygiene as unacceptable. Alia Al-Khalidi (2000) explains that the onset of menstruation for Victorian girls limited their already restricted participation in the public. Management and hygiene constrained Victorian women's education and communication to the home. Etiquette surrounding menstruation also meant that communication within the home was carefully negotiated and regulated.

Although menstruating women are not as radically confined to the private sphere, silence and verbal concealment of menstruation continues in elements of contemporary society. Al-Khalidi (2000) analyzed early advertising texts to reveal the public's distaste for the visibility and presence of menstruation and feminine hygiene products in American culture (Al-Khalidi, p. 67). Kissling (1996) argues that communication restrictions make up the core of the modern menstrual taboo, which is driven by "the belief that menstruation should not be talked about." Kissling explains:

> Menstruation must be concealed verbally as well as physically, and communication rules and restrictions permeate and define the concealment and activity taboos. A substantial majority of American adults and adolescents believe that it is socially unacceptable to discuss menstruation, especially in mixed company. Many believe that it is unacceptable to discuss menstruation even within the family.
> (Kissling, pp. 293–294).

Although the taboo confines menstruation to private discourse, it also generates pressure for a growing presence of and references to menstruation and feminine hygiene products in the mass media. Thus, Foucault's theory of the repressive hypothesis explains the simultaneous development of public restriction of menstruation "talk" and the extensive rhetorical devices in advertising to contain it. Discourses frame menses as an issue of private "hygiene." The idea that visible or public menstruation is threatening requires strict maintenance of women's hygiene and, though constrained, simultaneously *requires* the appearance of and talk about one's menses. In the same way that Victorians used specific contexts and discursive strategies to craft acceptable speech about sex, Americans accept the selling of feminine hygiene products to deflect public recognition of menstruation, justifying the modern explosion of "appropriate," public discourses surrounding menstrual products to further regulate any "threats." In short, we can trace the emergence of coded public discourse about menstruation to the creation of sanitary towels.

Al-Khalidi (2000) identifies 1880 as the year that material culture first began to market control of menstruation with the release of the first patent for the sanitary towel (p. 67). The product necessitated public discourse about the hygiene of menstruating women. Society tolerated such discourse because it primarily engaged management procedures, such as controlling the visibility of blood, eliminating the risk of odor, or obscuring other physical signs of menstruation. Analyzing advertisements for such items reveals that menstruation became a "public issue" only between the individual and the hygiene industry. To sustain the feminine hygiene industry market and capitalize on women's bodily processes to generate profit, menstruation needed to have a "public" presence, but discourse continued to control and police its advent. Not only did the acceptable discourses allow the consumer to adopt the illicit, metaphorical, and coded vocabularies, it also led consumers to purchase feminine hygiene products, like maxi pads and tampons, to police their bodies and control their menstruation.

Al-Khalidi's study shows that the catalogs that sold personal hygiene products further limited the products' visibility and encouraged the issue to remain a private topic by emphasizing discreetness. She argues that a "continuation of such strategies ... remains evident in contemporary consumption practices" (Al-Khalidi, 2000, p. 65). Likewise, Lee and Sasser-Coen (1996) emphasize that such practices of discipline and concealment are introduced to girls at an early age. This exposes them to "a plethora of subtle and not-so-subtle messages, whispered secretly in school playgrounds, stated matter-of-factly in lectures and documentaries, and boldly exclaimed in television commercials," and in some cases, "girls receive no direct personal information about menstruation at all" (Lee & Sasser-Coen, p. 61). These examples illustrate that explicit discourse in mainstream advertisements was concealed and repressed, while a coded proliferation of discourse simultaneously emerged. Discourse, which *should* relieve women of embarrassment and social anxiety and provide proper education on the subject of menses, instead remains limited and restricted. Such discursive trends encourage women to "hide menstruation, or else."

Examining discourses of popular culture, specifically those advertising feminine hygiene products, reveals that society perpetuates modern menstrual taboos through discursive strategies initiated and reinforced by pharmaceutical consumer industries. The present analysis illustrates, first, the ways in which Foucault's repressive hypothesis applies to regulating menstruation in the 21st century and, second, how patriarchy persists by regulating women's bodies to the private sphere and silencing voices on feminine issues.

One example of the repressed discourse of menstruation is found in an advertisement for Kotex Bodyfit Ultra Thin™ Sanitary Napkins (2004, p. 31). The print at the top explains: "Great news. But you can't hear it." The center of the advertisement contains a large sketch drawing of a young woman. The woman is drawn in shades of gray, and the woman's index finger is held up to her mouth, depicting the American hand gesture for "quiet." Since her lips are slightly parted, it looks as if she is quietly verbalizing the sound, "shhh." A red dot is found on the ring finger. The caption below the sketch reads: "Only Kotex® makes quiet pad wrappers. Less crinkling, less crackling. Because some things just aren't meant to be broadcast." The bottom right corner contains a picture of the product and the company motto: "Kotex® fits. Period."

The advertisement appeals to the tabooed belief that members of society should never know a woman is on her period. Although advertisements typically play on the fear of the sight of blood, this advertisement largely focuses on preventing the sounds now associated with periods. Recently, advertisements have begun emphasizing to women that, in addition to hiding and concealing their menstruation, they must also hide and conceal from the public the products and materials needed to cover up their menstruation. Houppert (1995) explains, "Forget the natural dismay of discovering you've bled through your skivvies to your skirt: these ads zeroed in on women's fear of exposure, promoting a whole culture of concealment. Tapping into that taboo, ads reinforced the idea that any sign that you were menstruating, even purchasing menstrual products, was cause for embarrassment" (p. 14). Additionally, advertisements remind women to conceal all products by highlighting plain wrappers and small sizes. Houppert (1996) continues, "the copy reminds readers how embarrassing it is to reach into a handbag for lipstick and pull out a tampon" (pp. 14–15). One advertisement published in multiple women's and teenage girl's magazines, including *Cosmopolitan* and *Seventeen,* in August 2007, symbolizes the need for women to hide signs of menstruation. The advertisement is printed on both sides of a magazine page. On the front of the advertisement, a 2 x 1½ size green box is centered in the middle of a white background. It reads, "Why be big if you don't have to be?" The o.b.® logo is located below the text, and the text beneath the logo reads: "mighty. small." On the back, the same size box, but turquoise-colored, appears in the center of the page surrounded by white background again. The text in the box reads: "Don't underestimate small. It can be pretty powerful. Take the o.b.® Tampon. It's designed small to protect big, expanding all-around to fit your shape perfectly. And with its new SilkTouch™ cover and Fluid-lock™ grooves for locked-in protection, this tiny tampon is as tough as it gets."

The message in this o.b.® advertisement plays upon the taboo that menstruating women should not show any sign of their menstruation. Rather than emphasizing the "leak" or the sound of "crinkling" wrappers, this advertisement also reminds women that wearing a pad, especially a large, bulging, and absorbent pad, risks society detecting your menstruation. It thus plays upon the taboo differently than the previous advertisements because it focuses attention on women's awareness that their pelvic area is perceptible and under public scrutiny. The advertisement claims that the best protection is found in *small*, yet absorbent, tampons.

Additionally, this advertisement emphasizes another social expectation: the ideal for young girls and women to remain thin. In our society, obesity is associated with feelings of shame and isolation, the same feelings equated with women who leak or show signs of menstruation publicly. Lee and Sasser-Coen (1996) argue that "such a discourse is especially aimed at teenagers, encouraging them to conceal bodily functions and keep their growing bodies small and thin lest they take up too much space, exercise power, or show evidence of failing in the disciplinary regimens of feminine bodily hygiene/care" (p. 60). Thus, girls are taught to associate the same pressures to maintain their weight with the social burdens placed upon them to preserve cleanliness and hygiene during their monthly period.

In the first advertisement, Kotex® furthers an ideology of concealment by emphasizing a woman's need to hide even the sound made by their feminine hygiene products. Because the most likely place to hear "crinkling" and "crackling" is in women's public restrooms, Kotex® tells consumers that such noises are inappropriate even in "private" spaces; secrecy becomes required even between women. Kotex® not only emphasizes the need for quiet products so as to not expose women using feminine hygiene products, but Kotex® also reinforces the belief that advertisements cannot openly discuss products and what they are designed to do without using coded language. In this instance, association of shame and secrecy remain primary messages.

Other print advertisements in this campaign are stylized and composed similarly and represent culturally diverse women. Some drawings change the skin tone and hair color to represent women of color. Through this depiction, Kotex® illustrates that the feeling of menstruation as an embarrassment and secret is a shared sentiment for all women regardless of ethnicity or race. The drawing also reinforces the taboo because the lips and the mouth are the only facial features drawn on the woman's face. The drawing does not contain eyes or a nose. The lack of features is another characteristic shared by all the drawings in this particular series of Kotex® advertisements. Featureless drawings may diminish the difference between the women, but in doing so, it represents the collective mentality that menstruation is taboo in Western culture regardless of race or ethnicity. Further, the lack of eyes and a nose is also symbolic, given that the taboo necessitates hiding the sight and smell of blood from the public.

In the Kotex® advertisement, coded discourse is apparent and enacted by the presence of the red dot, a socially sanctioned symbol for a woman's period. This advertisement conceals the obvious terminology of menstruation by replacing language largely with symbols. Rather than using the word "menstruation," the dot (creatively placed to represent a stone on a ring) is colored red in order to symbolize a literal red "period." The elimination of words reinforces the hidden and private nature of menstruation. According to Richard Weiner (2004), Kotex® achieved recognition in 2000 when it first featured the red dot in an advertisement to symbolize a woman's period (p. 27). Today, the red dot is used in most magazine ads and network TV commercials and has become a graphic icon. The word "period" also exists in this advertisement, but in this instance it is a play on words and contains a double meaning. Thus, rather than directly using the term *period* in the context of menstrual blood, it is used to emphasize the claim that "Kotex® fits." The obscured presence of "Period" indicates that the motto enacts the very strategy it advertises. Garfield (2000) further reifies the taboo by praising Kotex's® creative use of the word "period" and the red punctuation mark and by maintaining that the symbols and euphemisms go far enough.

He states: "All the stilted talk about "freshness" and all the blue-dye demos in the world fail to get to the point. By the same token, any more graphic use of the color red probably would be too much to stomach. So, in the realm of venturing into new frontiers, the colored punctuation mark is precisely far enough" (Garfield, 2000, p. 41). Reviews, like Garfield's, provide insight into the vicious cycle of the menstrual taboo: The industry does not use words and graphics that may offend their audiences and consumers, yet it is the continual usage of euphemisms and codes that instruct citizens to keep menstruation a private matter.

Advertisements for Procter & Gamble products further employ rhetorical proofs such as fear appeals as shown through a print advertisement that first appeared in *Cosmopolitan* in 2005. The advertisement consists of a photograph of a giant shark following a scuba diver. "A leak can attract unwanted attention" is the predominant caption. The terms *menstruation* and *period* are not stated, but the "leak" remains a reference to the menstrual cycle to women. "Leak," though ambiguous, is a common, alternative word understood as an acceptable synonym in the public discourse. In most advertisements in women's magazines, "leak" either refers to menstrual blood or urine. Women must look for other "clues" in the advertisement to determine which feminine hygiene product the advertisement is promoting. In this particular advertisement, a small picture of a box of Tampax Pearls™ appears in the bottom, right corner; however, the box does not contain the word "tampon." According to Lee and Sasser-Coen (1996) such equation of products with brands is not uncommon in the feminine hygiene industry. Often, women receive literature and information on menstruation from product companies that use their product's specific name interchangeably with hygiene supplies generally, furthering the ability of companies to eliminate and substitute discourse while also regulating products and practices on women's bodies. In addition to contributing to corporate capitalism, "this product-related information functions as a kind of 'propaganda,' and plays an important part in molding behavior and disciplining the body" (Lee & Sasser-Coen, p. 66).

The most significant element of the advertisement is its message, which tells women that "leaking" blood is not without consequences, being often dangerous and having deadly consequences. It plays upon the rumored misconception that leaks of blood can cause harm by attracting dangerous and deadly wild animals. According to Houppert, sources, like Harry Finley, curator of the Museum of Menstruation located in New Carrollton, Maryland, have disproven the myth that predators such as sharks and bears are attracted to the odor of menstruation. Houppert states: "Sound scientific documentation supporting such gender-biased malarkey is hard to find," he reports. "Actually, one is more likely to run across studies concluding quite the opposite" (Houppert, 2000, p. 211). Houppert also cites a 1991 article in the *Journal of Wildlife Management* that reports the results of studies conducted by the U.S. Forest Service. In the studies, bears consistently ignored used tampons and menstruating women (Houppert, pp. 211–212). Despite this research, an assumption remains implicit in the advertisement: metaphorically, leaks are equivalent to social death.

The Tampax Pearl™ Tampon advertisement is also significant because of its symbolism. First, the entire advertisement contains shades of the color, blue, and second, the advertisement pictures ocean water. Both the color blue and the image of water represent a sense of cleanliness and purity. Additionally, the color red is eliminated from the advertisement to encourage women to hide their menstruation from the public and to indicate that the use of tampons will assure such concealment. Thus, women are encouraged to buy tampons because they associate the cleanliness and hiding their blood with application of the tampon.

Other advertisements for Tampax Pearl™ Tampons emphasize more "realistic" scenarios where leaking blood and exposing menstruation are likely to have social consequences. Two advertisements show women engaging in activities that are traditionally viewed as unsafe and risky for menstruating women's participation. The first advertisement, which appeared in *Glamour* in 2006, shows a crowded party scene. A young woman is sitting on the shoulders of a young man. She looks comfortable, happy, and confident. She is wearing white pants. The second advertisement, found in *Jane* in May 2007, shows a woman on a diving board preparing to dive. She is wearing a white bathing suit. The text on the advertisement exclaims, "The braid makes you brave." The caption in small, white print reads "Only Pearl gives you trusted Tampax® protection and a revolutionary leak-catching braid."

In these particular advertisements, the menstruating woman is portrayed as naturally unconfident. Thus, in order to maintain her confidence and social status, a woman must engage in proper hygiene and purchase the best product for hiding signs of menstruation. These advertisements are particularly interesting because, in one way, they appear to disprove the tabooed message that women cannot participate in the public sphere and engage in behaviors if they are menstruating. Even though the advertisements display women "freed" from the taboo's restrictions, they also reinforce it by implying that the menstruating woman is only permitted in the public sphere with the correct hygiene and menstrual products; *naturally*, the menstruating woman does not belong and cannot employ the same level of participation. In this instance, a message is sent that women must control their bodies. Women learn to "pass" in public so that they can meet their culture's norms and expectations. Such menstrual politics reference the ideas in the early 20th century when women were restrained from physical sports "because their menstrual blood might 'stain' the playing fields" (Delaney, Lupton, & Toth, 1971, p. 55). Thus, by showing a woman, specifically a woman wearing a white bathing suit, the advertisement appears progressive because it sets aside an old-fashioned belief surrounding menstruation. However, in order to sell its product, Tampax® needs to maintain the fundamental belief that knowledge of menstruation is socially harmful. Hygienic gate-keeping procedures must occur prior to entering the public sphere. If they do not, women will be condemned to isolation and the private sphere because menstruation cannot be made public.

In the o.b.® Tampons advertisement, referenced above, codes and symbols are used to obfuscate other messages potentially dangerous to women. For example, the graphic of a small box of o.b.® tampons is more evidence that a trend exists to equate a particular brand with a product and to avoid using the words "menstruation" and "period." Additionally, the white space surrounding small boxes remains "unstained" and pure. The colors of the boxes are light green and turquoise and contain images of plants and flowers. Together, the colors and decorative prints portray o.b.® Tampons as natural and healthy. Until recently, due to the introduction of all-cotton tampons, tampon usage has been linked to toxic shock syndrome (TSS), a potentially fatal disorder that occurs in a disproportionate number of menstruating women and the increase of dioxin levels in women's bodies (Houppert, 1995, pp. 13–40). However, advertisements, like that for o.b.® tampons, use symbols, colors, and codes to overcome the fear of health risks from tampon usage and instead emphasize the fears and threats that accompany visibility of menstruation. Houppert (1995) explains:

> In most ways, the menstrual products industry is like any other. It plays on women's insecurities—Am I leaking? Will this pad show?— and develops ad campaigns to maximize these fears. Where it departs from mainstream corporate culture is in the secrecy that permeates every aspect of the business. Promising the invisibility of its products, it carries that commitment into its factories and boardrooms, cultivating a low profile that precludes public scrutiny. (p. 36)

The rhetorical analyses of the advertisements show that women are taught specific, negative associations to menstruation through the medium of print advertisements. Despite the integration of liberal feminist ideologies, today's feminine hygiene products like Playtex still play on the same insecurities developed in the early 20th century (Houppert, 1995, p. 37). Rhetorical readings of print advertisements reveal that reoccurring themes of shame, secrecy, social exclusion, dirtiness, and leakiness are consistently found in contemporary advertising campaigns.

Not only do these messages affect the way women relate to their body, but they also have serious and dangerous implications for women. For example, fear appeals in advertising persuaded women to purchase products that were physically harmful and deadly. According to Houppert (1995), in 1980 alone, 38 women died of TSS. These deaths correlated with the introduction of Rely, Procter and Gamble's most absorbent brand of tampons to hit the market. That same year, Houppert (1995) explains, Procter and Gamble (P&G) mailed 60 million free samples of Rely to consumers across the country. As the popularity of the product spread and the Centers for Disease Control reflected on the increased number of cases of TSS since 1979 (55 deaths and 1066 cases of nonfatal TSS), the center took note that the cases tended to occur primarily in young menstruating women. Soon after, studies and investigations revealed the connection between tampons and TSS. Although medical and scientific studies indicated that all major brands of tampons are associated with TSS, the National Academy of Sciences cited four studies that showed a correlation between the use of Rely and an increased risk of toxic shock (Slade & Biddle, 1982). Shortly thereafter, in September 1980, P&G removed Rely from the market.

According to Houppert (1995), Rely was "made of superthirsty synthetics such as carboxymethylcellulose and polyester" and "was billed as the most absorbent tampon ever to hit the market" (p. 29). Exacerbated by P&G's neglect of consumer complaints[2] and the FDA's lack of testing and labeling requirements for the industry,[3] women became victims of the feminine hygiene industry's profits. Because of the ongoing menstruation taboo, TSS remains an identifiable and negotiated risk to most young women who wear tampons. More importantly, TSS is still relevant because it illustrates that consequences occur when advertising campaigns scare consumers into purchasing products for maintaining social etiquette while downplaying the product's actual dangerous and potentially deadly effects. Even though TSS is now a commonly recognized risk, the misinformation or lack of information surrounding menstruation and the menstruation taboo continue to leave young girls at risk of physical harm.

Recent scientific studies suggest that tampon use not only puts women at risk of TSS, but also exposes women to high trace levels of dioxins. If dioxin toxins are building in women's bodies at a faster rate due to tampon use, women may risk hormonal changes that are medically linked to decreased fertility, ovarian dysfunction, and endometriosis (Houppert, 1995, p. 23). Houppert (1995) notes that concern about dioxin has not yet sparked consumer outrage. She explains that this is further evidence that "the code of silence surrounding menstrual hygiene leaves consumers with little information and less clout" (Houppert, p. 28). Lack of open communication about menstruation and feminine hygiene products as well as the emphasis on fear appeals is a dangerous discursive combination because it leads to negative material effects on women's bodies, such as illness and even death. Thus, the desire to eliminate all evidence of menstrual blood and the negative social effects of menstruation described in advertisements are most likely continuing to expose women to bodily harm.

Conclusion

Examining the current discourses surrounding menstruation first illustrates that surveillance, normalization, and agents of control are more present in the lives of women than men. The attempts to repress menstruation are directly linked to issues of power and gender politics. Even though society's understanding of menstruation appears less taboo, coded discourses surrounding menstrual products proliferates throughout our culture. Talk surrounding menstruation appears everywhere, yet educated and frank discussions about women's bodies are continually sanctioned to the private sphere (or even discouraged entirely).

Coded discourse, euphemisms, symbols, metaphors, and the erasure and avoidance of certain words produce attitudes toward menstruation that spill over to affect our assumptions of women and their bodies. Colors are also symbolic, and graphics and pictures often contain shameful, secret ,and deadly undertones. Additionally, the absence or elimination of certain words, such as "menstruation," reinforces the idea that menstruation is a taboo occurrence that must be carefully regulated and controlled in the public sphere. Social discourse surrounding menstruation, as shown in feminine hygiene product advertisements, reveals the reinforcement of taboo messages: Women are naturally leaky, women are dirty and dangerous to themselves, and women must strive to hide/silence all signs of menstruation.

Discursive trends and formations surrounding menstruation produce three consequences. First, women's bodies, their natural processes, and bodily hygiene remain confined to the private sphere and cause women to succumb to hegemonic cultural norms. By keeping menstruation and the enactment of hygiene private through coded discourse, Western culture discursively maintains the contemporary taboo and restricts women's social advancement. Such silencing and embarrassment concerning women's bodies and bodily acts will also likely limit women's voices and their willingness to discuss health-related issues surrounding their reproductive system and menstrual cycle in other spheres, such as in the medical community.

Second, outside of the occasional commercial or print advertisement, some men and women still completely avoid and/or silence positive and educational voices about menstruation in the public sphere. Limiting discussions risks the physical health and emotional well-being of girls and women who may incorrectly use tampons or live their lives feeling victimized and ashamed due to their menstrual cycle.

Third, the shift in the menstruation taboo from one that affects the public to one that affects women's personal interests appears to coordinate with the emergence of mass-produced feminine hygiene products and their consumption. Although the creation of feminine hygiene products helped women access the public sphere, the way in which products are sold today still subtly maintains the taboo and feelings of shame, anxiety, embarrassment, and fear. This may be more dangerous because the mass media appear to promote an open, public discourse while actually sanctioning the particular topic. Although discourse appears better than silence or erasure, Foucault argues that repressive discourse is just as harmful and potentially more dangerous because people engage in the discourse thinking that their discourse contains emancipatory potential when it does not. Thus, I have shown how repressed discourse acts as a strategy used by the mass media to maintain a taboo, successfully selling products to help women control menstruation, a "problem" that no one appears to discuss openly. Like other forms of patriarchy, the menstrual taboo is a taught, societal symptom.

The lack of open and direct discussion of menstruation, hygiene, and menstrual products allows the continuation of myths, taboos and dangerous health risks, threatening the safety of women. As long as aspects of the taboo confine women's bodies and hygiene to the private sphere and silence explicit, educated voices and discourse, the menstruation taboo will assert biopolitical control over women's bodies and potentially lead to deadly effects.

Notes

1. Multiple menstruation taboos exist throughout the world, and taboos also vary in Western cultures. This chapter provides examples of dominant messages, which characterize a range of Western menstruation taboos, but ultimately examines the contemporary hegemonic messages surrounding menstruation found in American culture.
2. On an average, P&G received 177 consumer complaints about Rely during each month it was on the market. Although not all of the complaints centered on the connection of TSS with Rely, the corporation instructed salespeople and marketers to deny "any link between tampons and toxic shock" (Houppert 30).
3. The FDA failed to require tampon manufacturers to label warnings on the side of the box, nor did it standardize ranges of absorbency (Houppert 31).

References

Al-Khalidi, A. (2000). "The greatest invention of the century:" Menstruation in visual and material culture. In M. Andrews & M. M. Talbot (Eds.), *All the world and her husband: Women in the twentieth-century consumer culture* (pp. 65–81). London: Cassell.

Bullough, V. L., & Bullough, B. (1995). *Sexual attitudes: Myths and realities.* New York: Prometheus.

Crawford, P. (1981). Attitudes to menstruation in seventeenth-century England. *Past and Present, 91,* 47–73. Retrieved November 1, 2012, from http://www.jstor.org.

Delaney, J., Lupton, M. J., & Toth, E. (1971). *The curse: A cultural history of menstruation.* New York: Mentor.

Foucault, M. (1978). *The history of sexuality: Volume 1.* Trans. R. Hurley. London: Penguin.

Garfield, B. (2000). Finally a feminine hygiene ad gets straight to the point. *Advertising Age, 71,* 41. Retrieved June 18, 2005, from http://web.ebscohost.com.

Houppert, K. (1995). *The cure: Confronting the last unmentionable taboo: Menstruation.* New York: Farrar.

Kissling, E. A. (1996). 'That's just a basic teen-age rule': Girls' linguistic strategies for managing the menstrual communication taboo. *Journal of Applied Communication Research, 24,* 292–309. Retrieved June 18, 2005, from http://web.ebscohost.com.

Kotex. (2004, December). [Advertisement for bodyfit ultra thin™ sanitary napkins.] *Health*, 31.

Laqueur, T. (1990). *Making sex: Body and gender from the Greeks to Freud*. Cambridge, MA: Harvard University Press.

Lee, J., & Sasser-Coen, J. (1996). *Blood stories: Menarche and the politics of the female body in contemporary US society*. New York: Routledge.

Martin, E. (1987). *The woman in the body: A cultural analysis of reproduction*. Boston: Beacon.

Niccoli, O. (1990). Menstruum Quasi Monstruum: Monstrous births and menstrual taboo in the sixteenth century. (M. A. Galluchi, M. M. Galluchi & C. C. Galluchi, Trans.) In E. Muir & G. Ruggiero (Eds.), *Sex and gender in historical perspective* (pp. 1–25). Baltimore, MD: Johns Hopkins University Press.

o.b. (2007, July). [Advertisment for o.b. tampons.] *Cosmopolitan*, n.p.

Procter and Gamble. (2005, July). [Advertisement for Tampax Pearl Tampons.] *Cosmopolitan*, 221.

Procter and Gamble. (2006, April). [Advertisement for Tampax Pearl Tampons.] *Glamour*, n.p.

Procter and Gamble. (2007, May). [Advertisement for Tampax Pearl Tampons.] *Jane*, n.p.

Rierdan, J., & Hastings, S. A. (1990). *Menstruation: Fact and fiction. Center for Research on Women, Working Paper No. 216*. Wellesley, MA: Wellesley College.

Slade, M., & Biddle, W. (1982, June 6). Ideas and trends in summary; New findings on toxic shock. *The New York Times*, p. 8. Retrieved November 1, 2012, from http://www.lexisnexis.com.

Weiner, R. (2004, July). A candid look at menstrual products—Advertising and public relations. *Public Relations Quarterly*, 26–28. Retrieved June 18, 2005, from http://web.ebscohost.com.

12 Voicing Women's Abortion Stories within Larger Cultural Narratives

Jamie L. Huber

Introduction

Given its cultural stigma, abortion is a topic that is often surrounded by silence, leaving women's voices about their abortion experiences unheard and their stories untold. Creating multiple spaces for women to share their stories and abortion experiences is an extremely important goal. These stories should play a significant role in shaping reproductive health policies, as well as cultural narratives about reproduction. I came to collecting abortion narratives and doing reproductive justice-based research as an activist and options counselor, and then as a researcher. In many ways I went through women's experiences with them as their stories were in progress. As a result, I became interested in collecting and researching these stories.

In this chapter, I utilize narratives collected from 14 women of varying backgrounds, all of whom are identified by pseudonyms. The narratives explore the abortion experience and the ways in which facets of identity (race, class, age, etc.) impact both that experience and broader reproductive health experiences for these women, tying them to broader sociocultural and sociohistorical ideologies. At times, these narratives complement one another. At other times, they contradict one another. Sometimes there are even discrepancies within one woman's individual narrative.

Women, for a variety of reasons, might construct their abortion experiences in very different ways. These constructions about abortion can include the emotional aspects, the physical aspects, the decision-making process, the influence of one's social support system, and reflections on having the abortion. However, even if their abortion experiences are constructed differently, there might be underlying themes that link these women's stories and experiences together. The women I interviewed often spoke of shame, self-blame, fear, apprehension, guilt, panic, and despair. These were common themes that seemed to bridge their experiences. Still, some differences among their experiences emerged. Some women were very conflicted about their decisions to have abortions; others were not. Some women saw the decision to have an abortion as an act of agency and empowerment; others did not. For some women, their sense of morality and spirituality was a significant factor in their decision-making process or their coping process. For others, it was not. Some women believe their abortions were great decisions, others found relief in their abortions but preferred not think about them, and others regretted their decisions.

Even though these women's constructions of their experiences differ owing to the shared abortion experience, these narratives are inextricably linked to one another. Although these women's constructions of their experiences can be very interesting, informative, and telling in themselves, it's important to remember that they occur in a greater context that shapes the ways in which these women viscerally experience, perceive, and tell their own stories. Cara J. MariAnna (2002) defines cultural narratives as "those stories that articulate cultural norms," and she goes on to quote Laurel Richardson, who states: "They are told from the point of view of the ruling interest and the normative order. As such, cultural stories maintain the status quo" (qtd. in MariAnna, pp. xvii–xviii).[1]

The narratives my interviewees have shared fit into larger cultural narratives in a variety of ways: as cautionary tales, as narratives of agency and self-empowerment and of power and privilege, as stories of social support and as tales of self-expression. I seek to present a deeper analysis of the ways in which these narratives function and fit together as pieces of these larger cultural narratives and to address the importance of, as well as the strategies for, bringing the stories of real women's lived experiences to these cultural narratives.

Cautionary Tales

In some ways, the abortion narratives function as cautionary tales. They are stories of what happens to women and girls when they are "too careless," or in Aurora's case,[2] the story can serve as a cautionary tale about abortion itself. Although they do not go about it in an explicit manner, the women themselves also construct their narratives as cautionary tales. As narrators, many of the women make statements that participate in such a construction, particularly when discussing both the shame associated with an unplanned pregnancy and an abortion, and the hardships they faced when attaining one. Lori comments that she "knew better" but was just "careless," and Emilie states that she "was stupid" and "just shouldn't have had sex." In a similar vein, Cheryl shares that "Maybe I would've been a little smarter had I had something to go on to try to keep myself safe. Then maybe I wouldn't have had to have the abortion." Valerie also says that, had she been better educated about safe sex, she might have avoided the unplanned pregnancy altogether. She goes on to remark on the distress the pregnancy and proceeding abortion caused her and her family. Cumulatively, these stories can function as a warning to girls and young women who engage in sexual activity outside of marriage. In U.S. culture, girls and young women are often warned about the dangers of having premarital sex, including tainting one's morality, ruining one's reputation, shaming one's family, pregnancy, and sexually transmitted infections. These are prevalent stereotypes and assumptions, even though, as Anna's story[3] shows, being happily married does nothing to magically protect a woman from an ill-timed pregnancy. Although the women I interviewed did not explicitly reference any cultural narrative, each woman definitely constructed her story in ways that play into the narrative of a cautionary tale.

Delia[4] and Aurora's abortion narratives function as cautionary tales in different ways. Although Delia is very content with her decision to have an abortion, the negative physical experience she had during the abortion plays into the cultural conception of abortion as a horrific, dangerous experience that harkens back to pre-*Roe v. Wade* days. Even though these extreme horror stories are exceptionally rare in contemporary society, the outlying horror story (like Delia's) continues to contribute to the cultural narrative of the horror of abortion and the ways in which abortion can hurt women—a narrative on which the anti-abortion movement heavily relies. Aurora's abortion narrative also plays into this cultural narrative, though the impact of her abortion experience is more psychological and emotional than physical. The amount of regret she displays over her decision to have an abortion constructs the aftermath of an abortion as a horrifying experience, and one that is harmful to women, again playing into the "abortion as horror" cultural narrative that is so prevalent in the anti-abortion rhetoric.

The abortion narratives I collected serve as cautionary tales in different ways. They might function as a cautionary tale against premarital sex; as a cautionary tale about the dangers of inadequate sex education; as a cautionary tale against "naively" trusting doctors, pharmacists, or various methods of pregnancy prevention; or as a cautionary tale against abortion itself. In many instances, the narratives function in congruence with a larger cultural narrative that reinforces the chastity of young women. Although most of my interviewees do not necessarily adhere to this larger cultural narrative, it still informs us about how they construct their experiences of unplanned pregnancy and abortion. No matter the specific tale, however, there is a rhetorical value for the teller that goes beyond simply sharing her experience for the sake of others, or self-expression. Cautionary tales imply that the teller has learned something, which serves as a form of recovery of her own agency, for the purpose of self-empowerment. However, when the agency takes the form of "self-disciplining" of inappropriate sexuality, such lessons become harder to celebrate. This theme of agency is more explicitly developed in some of the women's stories, as I will discuss in the following section.

Narratives of Agency and Self-Empowerment

Agency is a prominent theme among the narratives of the women I interviewed, and this theme interacts with larger cultural narratives in interesting and complex ways. With the exception of Cheryl,[5] all of the women I interviewed claimed agency over their decisions to have abortion. Even

Cheryl claimed this agency to some extent, though her circumstance due to her age and the wishes of her family was much more pressured. By making statements such as "I knew what I had to do," "I did what I needed to do for myself," and "I made the best choice for me," the women construct their abortions as events over which they had agency, and through that agency found self-empowerment in what often seemed demoralizing situations. Such agency and empowerment are extremely important in maintaining these women's psychological well-being and become particularly important for women like Emanda[6] and April,[7] who had been actively and "responsibly" engaging in behaviors to prevent pregnancy. With an unplanned pregnancy, a sense of control over one's own body and life is in some ways lost, as indicated by my interviewees' commenting on the extent to which they panicked upon learning they were pregnant. Cultural narratives about the duty of motherhood and the self-sacrificing mother abound, and in a sense, by claiming their agency and looking to themselves and their own needs instead of those of an unborn "child," these women defy that narrative.

In claiming agency and self-empowerment, most of these women also defy the cultural narrative that women are not able to make choices for themselves and do not know what is best for them. The antichoice movement often draws upon this cultural narrative, claiming that because women are unable to make hard life decisions for themselves, the abortion service industry exploits them. The idea behind this narrative is that women are more or less tricked into having abortions and will afterward face deep regret and sorrow that will haunt them for the rest of their lives. As I stated, most of the women I interviewed defy this narrative. Aurora's story, however, is very much in line with this narrative. Although Aurora made a logical decision to have an abortion owing to her financial situation, she has come to believe she was mistaken in that decision. Although she does not necessarily believe she was tricked into this decision, she does—at least to some extent—believe she was misled. She relays this idea when she speaks of how supportive her friends were of her decision, and how she wishes they had not been. Although she recognizes that her friends were well intentioned, she believes they gave her a false sense of security about the morality and acceptability of her having an abortion. She has also experienced a tremendous amount of regret regarding her decision, as evidenced by her continual attempts to seek forgiveness.

Among the women I interviewed (Aurora and Cheryl), Aurora is the only one whose story is part of the cultural narrative of abortion exploiting women. Aurora's story is still more nuanced than the cultural narrative itself. Cheryl, who at times experiences substantial concern about having an abortion, does not really fit into this cultural narrative. Although Cheryl did not have a great deal of agency or empowerment in her decision, she does not view herself as having been exploited, and she recognizes that the decision was ultimately in her own best interest.

Although some of the women I interviewed might experience occasional grief or sorrow as a result of their abortion, they generally claim the experience to have been an empowering one, in which they were able to express at least some degree of agency in a situation in which they felt quite powerless. This agency and self-empowerment in many ways defies many cultural narratives, particularly those that present an ideal of self-sacrificing motherhood, as well as those that claim abortion exploits women. However, some women, including one of my interviewees in particular, have experiences that are more in line with the aforementioned cultural narratives, and they therefore downplay either their own agency in the abortion process or any empowerment associated with the decision to have an abortion.

Stories of Social Support

The importance and influence of social support was evident among the narratives of the women I interviewed, making this a central theme that intertwines the women's various accounts of their abortion experiences. When negotiating the abortion process, several women I interviewed sought solace from their family and friends, as one might expect. After all, "family and friends" cultural scripts suggest that one should seek comfort from friends and family when going through a stressful life event. Still, some of my interviewees were, for a variety of reasons, not able to seek support from family or friends, creating a disjunct between their own, personal narratives and larger cultural narratives. This paradox left these women seeking support in less traditional places.

Although some women did receive the support of family and friends that traditional cultural scripts dictate, several of the women did not. Disapproval from family, disapproval from friends, abusive relationships, and living in a different country than one's family and friends kept some women from seeking this type of social support. Sometimes, as in cases of disapproval and particularly abusive relationships, "support" from loved ones was rhetorically constructed as more harmful than helpful, as in the cases of both Delia[8] and Cally.[9] These narratives resist the cultural scripts that construct family and friends as positive sources of social support. In apparent recognition of the rhetorical power of others' viewpoints, then, several women sought to isolate themselves from their usual support networks in order to protect their own agency.

Rather than having supportive family and friends, some women had to turn to other places. Several women found unforeseen kindness and support in strangers, which could include the clinic staff. Most notable was Jennifer, who welcomed support from staff at a women's shelter when she found herself unexpectedly pregnant, in an abusive relationship, and in a foreign country far away from her friends and family. Those who find support among strangers, particularly when they are unable to find support among friends and family, defy the cultural narratives and expectations of social support. Still, the powerful potential of social support, regardless of its source and valence, was a consistent theme among the narratives of the women I interviewed.

Tales of Self-Expression

For some of the women I interviewed, telling me their stories seems to have been a way for them to express themselves and gain a sense of catharsis, perhaps even validation. Yolanda, for example, had sought out counseling services so that she could talk about her abortion experience. Talking about her experiences was very helpful to her, giving her a cathartic release and a way to deal with some of her pent-up emotions. During our interview, she told me that speaking with me and talking about her experience was therapeutic, just as her counseling sessions were. Similarly, Aurora stated that talking about her experience helped her come to terms with her actions, and aided her on her road to forgiveness. For both of these women, being able to tell their stories was an important part of their process of dealing with their abortions.

Even several of the women I interviewed who did not necessarily desire to tell their stories as a way of dealing with their abortion experiences still appreciated the opportunity to tell their stories. April commented, "It's refreshing to talk to someone about this in such an open way," and Lydia stated, "I've enjoyed being able to talk with you." Emanda shares, "Even though I feel removed from the experience now, I think it's good to think about it sometimes and talk about my experience. I actually think there should be a lot more women talking about their experiences. Then when we go through all of it we won't feel so alone and isolated." These comments fit into a larger social notion about the need for catharsis and self-expression, as well as the cultural narrative that everyone has a story to share. So self-expression becomes rhetorically constructed as an opportunity for healing and connection. However, as Emanda states, not everyone shares her story.

With her comment, Emanda taps into the reality that in U.S. culture, as well as others, abortion narratives are often silenced or taboo. Such silencing creates a culture in which women who are seeking an abortion often face feelings of shame, isolation, and loneliness. So although many women can find points of connection among their stories and experiences, they remain disconnected from one another. This silencing also makes it more difficult for women to negotiate the process of attaining an abortion, particularly for immigrant women like Yolanda and Jennifer, because fewer resources exist for them to consult. Various campaigns are attempting to remedy this silencing of abortion, such as: Jennifer Baumgardner's "I Had an Abortion" campaign, imnotsorry.net, Project Voice's theabortionproject.org, the Abortion Conversation Project, and Backline's "The Abortion Diaries." Still, a great deal more work needs to be done in this area, as the cultural narrative enforcing silence around issues of sex and abortion is particularly entrenched.

Narratives of Privilege and Power

In addition to the cultural narratives mentioned above, the narratives of the women I interviewed are also part of larger cultural narratives, and discourses, of privilege and power. These specific stories fit into cultural narratives and discourses in a variety of ways, particularly as they draw upon issues of race, nationality, income, geographic location, and power differentials within an actual abortion clinic setting. It is at these points of identity and their intersections that Critical Race Feminism is made most relevant.

Hypersexualization

Several of my interviewees discussed race as a significant factor in their experiences of abortion. Two of my interviewees, for example, explicitly critiqued the stereotypes of their races as hypersexualized. This stereotype comes from a larger cultural discourse that constructs ethnic minority women as hypersexualized and animalistic. This is a discourse that one can see played out in a variety of arenas, perhaps most notably in advertisements where ethnic minority women are often portrayed in seductive poses donning animal and jungle print lingerie (Merskin, 2010, p. 207). This stereotype also draws upon the notions that ethnic minority women are oversexed, always available for sex, "breeders," and "welfare queens" (Collins, 1990, pp. 84, 284). Societal perceptions about certain identity markers (such as race) and the ways in which they intersect with other identity markers (such as class) allow for the continued existence of this stereotype, as it builds upon the bases of both slavery and the eugenics movement. During slavery, Black women were viewed as property, including sexual property, and were expected to be available on command for various sexual acts and breeding purposes (Collins, 1990, pp. 125, 133). After Emancipation, the notion of Black women as sexual property continued to persist and be discursively re-created, and eventually morphed into today's cultural conception of hypersexualized ethnic minority women (Collins, 1990, pp. 129, 174). The eugenics movement also furthered the discursive re-creation of the hypersexualization of minority women with their fear-filled rhetoric that focused on how the "inferior" minority races would overtake the "superior" white race owing to their incessant breeding (Roberts, 1997, p. 60).

According to culturally dominant notions of femininity, a woman is supposed to be pure, pious, and domestic, so to be sexual—especially hypersexual—contradicts this notion of femininity (Shaw & Lee, 2009, pp. 432–433). This type of womanhood was reserved for refined women, or ladies, who were of "superior" class and racial status. Although this notion of femininity was an 18th-century ideal, remnants of it still exist within contemporary discourses. When women fail to meet this outdated ideal, particularly in terms of racial and class status, they can be understood by others as hypersexualized and as social aberrations. Referring to the way she perceives the doctor as constructing her as a woman who is of an inferior race and from an inferior class, and who has subpar intelligence, Lori comments of her doctor: "He was very condescending, and acted like I was just some hypersexualized girl from the ghetto who didn't have enough sense to use birth control." As such, he attempted to convince Lori to utilize more long-acting forms of birth control, despite her stated preference for pills, and then he went on to explain how to take the pill in excruciating detail, likely because he doubted Lori's ability to effectively take the pill. Although she does not use the term *hypersexualized* as Lori does, Lydia also indicates that her doctor constructed her as oversexed, presumably based on the way he interpreted her race and class, indicating that she needed to use long-lasting forms of birth control, and stating that purchasing a high-priced IUD would be cheaper than returning for multiple abortions, assuming that she would, indeed, return for multiple abortions. Like Lori, Jazmin also explicitly references being hypersexualized, though her reading of hypersexualization came not from the doctor but from the clinic protestors calling her a "Mexican whore." Still, regardless of the source, the same discourses and narratives of race, class, and sexuality come into play.

Relative social positioning and power are important aspects of how this construction of hypersexualization can occur. The doctors, for instance, are in a substantial position of power relative to their patients. In a way, this creates space for the doctors to rhetorically construct their patients as "less than," perhaps based on various identity aspects such as race and perceived class, if they so choose. Patients like Lori and Lydia can refuse doctors' insistent suggestions to take different types of birth control, and they might internally resist doctors' attempts to construct them in a certain way, but their outlets to externally resist the attempts are limited, particularly if they must rely on the doctors for services. Women who are depending on a doctor for an abortion physically and practically have more at stake than the doctor, giving the doctor more power to construct his or her patients as he or she will, with little consequence. Similarly, the protestors are also in a position of power relative to the patients, allowing them to construct abortion patients in whatever ways they choose, while facing little consequence. Although the protestors do not have professional credibility to grant them power, or the patients' reliance on their services, their bodies are not placed on the line as the bodies of the patients they confront are. By situating themselves in a confrontational role that draws upon the fact that the patients' bodies are already on the line, protestors place themselves in a position of power over the patients, and they also place themselves in a position that gives voice to their rhetorical constructions of the patients. Although the patients do not necessarily need to give any credence to these constructions, they still hear them as they are shouted out at them.

When faced with racist and classist constructions others are making of them, the women I interviewed expressed a variety of reactions. Lori, for instance, portrayed a substantial amount of anger, resentment, frustration, and disappointment with her doctor. She expressed these emotions when she stated, "I didn't want to have to explain myself to some jerk doctor." A woman going to a clinic for an abortion might logically presume that she is going to a pro-choice space and will be surrounded be staff who are supportive, helpful, and "on her side." For women like Lori, this presumption was soon shattered. When she made comments such as "some jerk doctor," she indicated disappointment in, as well as an antagonistic relationship with, the person who was supposedly helping her deal with the unplanned pregnancy. In actuality, the person was neither supportive nor trustworthy, at least in her eyes.

Lydia conveyed similar emotions when she spoke of her experience with her doctor. His continuous attempts to push unwanted forms of birth control on her caused her a great deal of frustration and resentment, particularly because she believes these attempts were based on her race. Even though Lori and Lydia resisted their doctors' constructions of them, they still had to yield to the doctors' directions when in the clinic space. Although Jazmin also portrayed some feelings of resentment and frustration toward the protestors who hypersexualized her, she focused on the event in a more casual manner and was, to some extent, bemused by what she called their ridiculous accusations. In this case, even though her body was on the line, she claimed a sense of agency in resisting the protestors' constructions of her. She was able to do this, in part, because she was not reliant upon the protestors and was not actually in their physical space.

Black Genocide

Another way in which race is made salient in some women's abortion experiences is through the rhetoric of "Black genocide," which is an oft-used rhetorical strategy of the anti-abortion movement. As a clinic escort, I have heard anti-abortion protestors yell the genocidal accusation of "You're killing your race" at Black women who entered the clinic. Similarly, Dázon Dixon (1990) tells of escorting a Black woman into a clinic while a young, blond, blue-eyed man screamed at her that Reverend Martin Luther King Jr. would "turn over in his grave for what *she* was doing" because she was contributing to her race's genocide. The woman turned to him and calmly said, "You're a White boy, and you don't give a damn thing about me, who I am or what I do. And you know even less about Martin Luther King or being Black. What you have to say to me means nothin', not a damn thing" (pp. 185–186). In this situation, this woman demonstrated how protestors use racialized rhetoric, and therefore racism, as a means to their own end in controlling women's reproduction. This theme was also brought out during my interview sessions, as Lori specifically referenced both protestors telling her she was killing her race and anti-abortion billboards in Georgia that utilized the "abortion is genocide" rhetoric.

When Lori spoke of the anti-abortion billboards, she referred to a billboard campaign that began in Georgia in February of 2011. At this time, several billboards were posted in Georgian communities that read, "Black Children Are an Endangered Species," and featured a photograph of an unhappy-looking Black child (Colb, 2010, para. 1). Although anti-abortion billboards are not uncommon, the provocative and racialized nature of these particular billboards sparked a great deal of controversy nationwide. Despite the controversy, the campaign spread, with similar sorts of billboards appearing across the country, in places such as Atlanta, New York, and Los Angeles. One of the billboards in New York, which has since been taken down, read, "The Most Dangerous Place for an African American Is the Womb." This billboard featured a young Black girl and became a point of contestation because the girl's mother was not told the purpose of the photos that appeared on the billboard (Kennedy, 2011, para. 2). Chenning Kennedy states that the discourses portrayed in these billboards "[have] tapped into a long and earned distrust among black Americans of the health care industry broadly. It trades on the real and troubling history of Planned Parenthood founder Margaret Sanger's early 20th century involvement with eugenics" (para. 2).

Sherry Colb (2010) analyzes the billboards in the context of Black incarceration, stating that the billboards play on the Black community's already existent fears of being endangered owing to the high percentage of Black individuals who face incarceration. According to Colb (2010), who cites the Bureau of Justice Statistics, the chances of a Black person going to jail in his or her lifetime are 18.4%, compared to 3.4% for a White person. Colb (2010) comments that "[r]acial disparities in incarceration, and perhaps in abortion as well, understandably trigger anger and discomfort in the African American community" (p. 2). As Colb (2010) states, although some might view the increased incarceration rates and abortion rights of Black Americans solely as issues of "personal responsibility," many might also view these as systemic issues, resulting from desolate situations. An increased incarceration rate, for example, can result from crimes being committed out of the disproportionate societal stress and poverty that many Blacks face, as well as "discretionary decisions by police and prosecutors about whether and how harshly to pursue different criminal suspects and defendants" (p. 3). Similarly, this disproportionate societal stress and poverty can also lead Black women to seek abortion services at a higher rate than White women do.

When discussing both the billboards and the issues involved with higher incarceration and abortion rates for Black individuals, Colb (2010) notes that opposing abortion is not a viable solution to remedy the situation of the Black community, even though the billboards "may inspire legitimate feelings of powerlessness and siege" (p. 4). When making suggestions that would help alleviate these deeper issues, Colb (2010) suggests a variety of societal steps that could be taken to address the issue of higher incarceration rates for Blacks, including: decriminalizing some of the offenses that consist of nonviolent activity, lessening the sentences for convictions based on nonviolent crimes, monitoring discretionary decisions by police and prosecutors in an effort to detect and punish racial bias, and addressing "the underlying concomitants of inner-city crime, including de facto segregation, poverty, and educational inequity ... thereby prevent[ing] crime through physical and emotional infrastructure" (p. 4).

Addressing the higher rates of abortion in the Black community would require a similarly complex approach, rather than simply adhering to a one-dimensional notion of opposing abortion, which would, in fact, actually exacerbate the problem of higher incarceration rates among Blacks. Opponents of abortion, such as the ones who created the "Endangered Species" billboards, seek to criminalize abortion, making women who seek abortion services, including Black women, criminals. Therefore, taking these billboards at face value and merely opposing abortion is not beneficial to the Black community.

Just as there are historically based sociocultural factors that lead to the stereotype of hypersexualized minority ethnic women, so are there historically based sociocultural factors that lead to actual increased incarceration and abortion rates among Blacks, as Colb (2010) so eloquently states. Anti-abortion groups can then play on these sociocultural factors in an attempt to induce fear and feelings of powerlessness in the Black community, placing Black women at the center of their campaign. It is at the intersections of gender, race, and class that Black women find themselves entangled in this situation. Because of the institutionalized poverty in many Black communities, Black women might choose to have an abortion out of economic need. It is then their status as women, and thereby potential carriers of fetuses, that positions them as targets of both the billboard campaign and the potential angry backlash. Since Black women who seek abortions are the "cause" of high rates of abortions in the Black community, the billboards directly confront them about their choices, urging them to consider that they are "killing their race" by choosing abortion and should therefore make a different choice. Additionally, the billboards have the potential to incite the Black community against Black women who choose to have abortions, considering them to be traitors to their race. The rhetorical construction of Black women who seek abortions being traitors to their race has roots in the Black Nationalist Movement and ultimately stems from the eugenics movement (Roberts, 1997, pp. 98–99). The anti-abortionists who created these billboards are seeking to capitalize on these connections to create abhorrence for abortion and those who seek abortions.

Of the women I interviewed, Lori was the only one who explicitly mentioned being told she was killing her race and who explicitly mentioned the "Endangered Species" billboard campaign. Still, the theme of Black genocide is a common one in the literature regarding both the experiences of women seeking abortions and anti-abortion rhetoric. It has also been a consistent theme and issue that Black women seeking abortions have had to deal with since at least the condemnation of abortion by the Black Nationalist Party, making this an important issue to address. Lori does not spend a great deal of time discussing the billboards or the comments that were yelled at her, mentioning them briefly as though they were ridiculous and hurrying past them as topics with an air of disgust. Yet she remembers them. Of all the comments protestors yelled at her, she specifically heard and remembered someone telling her she was killing her race. So the personal comments and public rhetoric she tried to present as personally inconsequential had a real impact on her and her body, just as it does on countless other Black women. When she speaks of her friends disagreeing with her decision to have an abortion,[10] and states that they think she is trying to be better than they are, perhaps they also disagree with her decision because in some way they too think she is killing her race. Whether or not that is true, it is a question that Lori might face. It is similar to the questions numerous Black women face when seeking abortion services, regardless of whether their race is ever explicitly called into question.

White Privilege and Colorblindness

An additional way in which narratives of privilege and power function in this study is through rhetorical constructions of colorblindness. As a child of the late 1980s/early 1990s, I grew up believing that a practice of colorblindness was ideal. I can still remember hearing En Vogue singing on the radio, "Free your mind and the rest will follow/Be colorblind, don't be so shallow." And of course, En Vogue was right. After all, who wants to be judged on the basis of their skin color? However, now that I am no longer a child, and it is no longer the 1980s or 1990s, I realize that a colorblind ideal is simple and problematic, and can by no means account for the complexities and nuances in real-life race relations. In many ways, the notion of colorblindness is the antithesis to Critical Race Theory and Critical Race Feminism. However, on many levels the colorblind ideal continues to persist in contemporary U.S. culture.

Although some might consider colorblindness a nice idea in theory, in practice it often serves to hide and thereby enable the mechanisms by which racism functions. A lens of colorblindness still maintains (already dominant) White sociocultural norms, while at the same time proliferating the idea that race does not matter and should be inconsequential. In reality, race remains consequential; years of racism and racialized social and political constructions and institutions have not been rendered nonexistent overnight. Rather, they still exist and White privilege becomes reinforced, even if done so on a covert level. So in a society promoting colorblindness, racism still exists. However, rather than existing in an explicit and overt manner, it comes to exist in implicit and covert ways, with the ideal of colorblindness hiding the very mechanisms that continue to reproduce it.

Colorblindness plays an important role in the narratives of my interviewees. Even the ethnic minority women I interviewed did not at first reference their race as part of their abortion experiences. They did not comment upon the racial aspects of their experiences until I specifically asked about race, thereby making it relevant. Until that moment, the research interview was operating in a colorblind framework, as colorblindness assumes we are living in a postracial society where race is no longer relevant. Interviewees can assume that I, as a White researcher who "does not have to deal with issues of race," do not think race is an important factor in women's abortion experiences. By specifically asking about race, I subvert the colorblind framework, allowing these women to more fully share their experiences. Still, these women are not often able to point to incidents of overt racism, with the few exceptions of slurs and comments yelled by anti-abortion protestors and the billboard campaign that Lori mentioned. Yet these women know they were somehow victims of racism, even though they cannot explicitly describe how. This conundrum is a result of colorblindness in practice; with few exceptions, race is not an overt factor in the abortion experience. However, racial bias and stereotypes are institutionalized, causing the treatment of these women potentially to be very different from the treatment White women might have. This is how colorblindness reproduces racism while at the same time hiding the existence of racism. Furthermore, colorblindness ignores the social conditions that create the demand for abortions among many minority women, as Colb alludes to when discussing the "Endangered Species" billboard campaign.

Even as colorblindness was an element in my interviews with ethnic minority women, it also played a prominent role in my interviews with White women. As a result of various identity factors, mostly class, geographic location, and age, the white women I interviewed were not in positions of extreme privilege. Many had financial issues, some were in geographically remote locations, and some were, or at least until recently, dependents. Yet they all had White privilege. When I asked the women to share their abortion experiences, they did not mention any aspects that were racial in nature. As I have mentioned, this was very similar to the ethnic minority women I interviewed. However, when I explicitly asked about race, the similarities ended. The White women did not view their race as having any impact on how they experienced their abortions. Yet by virtue of their perception that race is irrelevant (in contrast to the ethnic minority women's perceptions of race as relevant), the White women's race does rhetorically impact their experiences: *by allowing them to view it as inconsequential.* Again, this is how colorblindness covertly reinforces White privilege by centering White experiences as "the norm." In this light, even though women like Lori and Lydia have valid complaints regarding their treatment, they can be viewed as being oversensitive.

In summary, then, power and privilege are very important aspects of a woman's abortion experience, and these positions of power and privilege occur at the intersections of the woman's identity. Her race, class, age, geographic location, ability level, sexuality, and power relative to her doctor can all impact her experience, though some aspects of identity will impact her experience in more explicit ways than others. These discourses play into much larger cultural narratives of power and privilege, of the haves and the have-nots, and of how the have-nots should pull themselves up by their bootstraps. Most noteworthy, though, is how these discourses play into larger cultural narratives of who should have power and of whose experiences should be taken "as normal." Ethnic minority women who are hypersexualized and viewed as members of an "endangered species" are obviously not the norm.

Conclusion

In this chapter, I've discussed narrative themes that arose from my interviews. I examined how these narrative themes interact with various cultural narratives: Specifically, at times the themes reinforce the cultural narratives; at times the cultural narratives reinforce the themes; and at other times the themes defy the cultural narratives. Common ways in which the narratives I collected function are: as cautionary tales; as narratives of agency and self-empowerment; as stories of social support; as tales of self-expression; and as narratives of power and privilege. The cultural narratives often burden the women seeking abortions, or try to place them into boxes in which they do not fit. By constructing women who seek abortions, particularly ethnic minority women who seek abortions, in negative ways, many cultural narratives pose a threat to women and their agency. Problematic interactions with abortion providers, pharmacists who sell birth control, and abstinence-only sex education professionals confound these potential threats, as do women's financial situations. Given my research's grounding in Critical Race Feminism and reproductive justice, the narratives of privilege and power become particularly important, including the ways in which intersecting identity markers function. Although cultural narratives often function in threatening ways to women and their agency, at times they can actually be helpful, particularly those that encourage women's agency or the social support of women who are having abortions. Moreover, women can claim a great deal of agency by defying the cultural norms that, in all essence, are undermining them and their decisions. Unfortunately, the culture of silence surrounding abortion often limits and prohibits this agency. There are ways, however, to disrupt this silence, and the creation of both physical and virtual spaces where it is safe for women to share their stories is a great start.

Notes

1. See Richardson, L. (1988). "The collective story: Postmodernism and the writing of sociology." *Sociological Focus, 21*(2), 199–208.
2. While Aurora's Catholic upbringing only gave her slight pause when deciding to have an abortion, her later reconciliation with the Church has created a great deal of remorse and desire for forgiveness for her decision.

3. Anna and her husband were happily married and wanted children. However, their financial circumstances were not stable enough to grant them the ability to care for a child in the capacity they desired.
4. Delia faced poor clinic practice and hospitality, and had to go to the emergency room for treatment owing to abortion complications.
5. Cheryl was 13 at the time of her abortion and faced a great deal of pressure from her family to have the procedure.
6. Emanda's pharmacy switched her name brand birth control pill to a generic pill, which was less effective. Although she was taking the pill regularly, she still faced an unplanned pregnancy.
7. April was taking a birth control pill regularly and had an autoimmune disease that made the risk of pregnancy very unlikely. Still, she faced an unplanned pregnancy.
8. Delia's boyfriend, who faced mental health issues, made dealing with her abortion very emotionally taxing, as he oscillated from being very supportive and condemning her for the abortion.
9. Prior to her abortion, Cally had left her abusive husband, who was also a fundamentalist preacher. After her abortion, he continued to stalk her and try to persuade her to let him save her soul.
10. Lori spoke about her friends encouraging her to drop out of college so she could come home and raise her baby. They did not understand why she would want to have an abortion so she could continue her college education without any interruption.

References

Colb, S. F. (March 3, 2010). "Anti-abortion billboards claim 'Black children are an endangered species': A meaningful contention?" *FindLaw column*. Retrieved February 27, 2011, from: http://writ.news.findlaw.com/colb/20100303.html.

Collins, P. H. (1990). *Black feminist thought: Knowledge, consciousness, and the politics of empowerment*. New York: Routledge.

Dixon, D. (1990). "Operation oppress you: Women's rights under Siege." In M. G. Fried (Ed.), *From abortion to reproductive freedom: Transforming a movement* (pp. 185–186). Boston: South End Press.

Kennedy, C. (2011, February 28). "Is a black woman's womb a dangerous place?" *News for action*. ColorLines. Retrieved March 8, 2011, from: http://colorlines. com/archives/2011/02/is_a_black_womans_womb_a_...m_medium=feed&utm_campaign=Feed%3A+racewireblog+%28ColorLines%29.

MariAnna, C. J. (2002). *Abortion: A collective story*. Westport, CT: Greenwood.

Merskin, D. (2010). *Media, minorities, and meaning: A critical introduction*. New York: Peter Lang.

Roberts, D. (1997). *Killing the black body: Race, reproduction, and the meaning of liberty*. New York: Vintage Books.

Shaw, S. M., & Lee, J. (2009). *Women's voices, feminist visions: Classic and contemporary readings* (4th ed.). New York: McGraw-Hill, 2009.

Epilogue

Annette Madlock Gatison

Cultural and social norms are highly influential in shaping individual behavior that determines how we treat others and how we treat ourselves. These challenges to women's health create an atmosphere of expected conformity to those norms by some, whereas others might subscribe to those same norms, resulting in a culture of silence. I am pleased to have had the opportunity to present the work of scholars who use their position of privilege to advocate and allow the voices of women from a variety of racial, ethnic, and sociocultural backgrounds to have a say about their health. *Communicating Women's Health* helps to identify the social and cultural norms that keep women silent while providing ideas and strategies that seek to reshape those norms and provide voice.

Communicating Women's Health is an anthology that taps into the various cultural norms crossing the boundaries of age, race, class, ethnicity, and sexual orientation. Shifts and changes in cultural attitudes and expectations that have developed over decades and have been internalized can only be changed over time. However, drawing attention to issues such as depression, suicide, institutional racism, and media framing of health messages is only the beginning of a change in that dynamic, ranging from women being silent about their health to women voicing their concerns about their health. The discussions presented here regarding the social and cultural norms that impact women's health are only the tip of the iceberg on a vast continuum; many variables need to be considered and addressed by advocates, patients, healthcare providers, caregivers, and concerned others.

Contributors

Dr. Kimiko Akita is an Associate Professor in the School of Communication at the University of Central Florida, where she teaches international and intercultural communication, gender communication, and a cultural studies honors seminar in *manga* and *anime*. Dr. Akita publishes on gender communication, intercultural communication, international communication, media studies, pop culture, postcolonialism, and late capitalism. Her articles on gender and cross-cultural issues have appeared in journals and books, including *Global Media Journal*, *Women and the Media: Diverse Perspectives*, *Women and Language*, and the *Journal of Mass Media Ethics*. Dr. Akita earned her B.A. from Mount Mary College, Wisconsin; her M.A. in Communication-Urban Studies from Michigan State University; and her Ph.D. in Communication from Ohio University. Dr. Akita was a dissertation fellow at the Center's for Women's Intercultural Leadership at Saint Mary's College (University of Notre Dame) in Indiana, during 2002–2005.

Dr. Reynaldo Anderson currently serves as an Assistant Professor of Humanities at Harris-Stowe State University in Saint Louis, Missouri. Dr. Anderson has published articles and book chapters and has presented extensive research documenting the Africana experience and the Communication Studies field. For example, Dr. Anderson presented his latest research on the Africana futurist perspective at the Sorbonne in Paris, at a conference hosted by UNESCO. Dr. Anderson is a past chair of the Black Caucus of the National Communication Association. Finally, as an executive board member of the Missouri Arts Council, Dr. Anderson and other members procured resources from the American Recovery Act and utilized the stimulus to support the arts community in the region. Dr. Anderson was recognized in 2010 for his efforts in the humanities with a community leadership award from Governor Jay Nixon.

Dr. Andrée E. C. Betancourt is an independent interdisciplinary scholar and multimedia artist who has worked in the film industry. Dr. Betancourt received her Ph.D. in communication studies from Louisiana State University, and she was awarded a Graduate School Dissertation Fellowship for "Under Construction: Recollecting the Museum of the Moving

Image," a study that demonstrates ways in which we recollect our memories and ourselves through museum-going and technologies of reproduction. She taught courses across the communication discipline during her doctoral program and as an adjunct faculty member at the University of South Alabama in the Department of Communication. She received her B.A. in psychology from Smith College and her M.A. in film studies from University College Dublin. Currently a freelance writer and editor for a national consulting firm in the D.C. area, Dr. Betancourt has worked for numerous arts and cultural institutions in the United States and Europe. Her recent scholarship explores intersections among memory, collecting, and images (traditional and digital, moving and still), and she has presented her research at a number of conferences. Dr. Betancourt's essay "All about My Televisual Mothers: Talking Back to Carmela Soprano and Ruth Fisher" will be featured in the forthcoming anthology *Television and the Self: Knowledge, Identity and Media Representation.*

Dr. Andrea M. Davis is Assistant Professor of Communication Studies in the Department of Fine Arts and Communication Studies at University of South Carolina Upstate. Her research focuses on the performativity of space and gender, and health communication and sexuality. She earned her Ph.D. in Communication Studies and a graduate certificate in Women and Gender Studies from Bowling Green State University. She teaches communication theory, research methods, gender and communication, and health communication.

Elizabeth M. Davis (Ph.D., The Ohio State University) is an Associate Professor in the Department of Humanities and Communications at Embry-Riddle Aeronautical University in Prescott, Arizona. Dr. Davis' research explores the intersections where public, popular, and institutional discourses meet, conflict, and interact with individuals and with social practices. Her research has focused on risk communication, gender and health issues, medical discourse and identity, and the rhetoric of medicine. Her work as appeared in *Qualitative Health Research* and the *Journal of Applied Communication Research*. The author thanks the members of the Gonzaga Junior Faculty Interdisciplinary Writing Group, Rebecca Stephanis, Debra Hoover, Angela Beck, and Susan Bailie for their invaluable advice and support.

Dr. Sandra L. Faulkner is an Associate Professor of Communication at Bowling Green State University. Her teaching and research interests include qualitative methodology, poetic inquiry, and the relationships among culture, ethnic/sexual identities, and sexual talk in close relationships. She has published research in journals such as *Qualitative Health Research* and *Journal of Social and Personal Relationships*, and her books *Poetry as Method: Reporting Research through Verse* and *Inside Relationships: A Creative Casebook on Relational Communication* with Left Coast Press. Her poetry has appeared in *Qualitative Inquiry*,

Women and Language, Storm Cellar, Literary Mama, and *Northwoods.* Her chapbook, Hello Kitty Goes to College, was published by dancing girl press. She lives in northwest Ohio with her partner, their warrior girl, and a rescue mutt.

Dr. Manda V. Hicks is an Assistant Professor and Director of Forensics at Boise State University. She is an OEF/OIF veteran and former sergeant in the U.S. Army. Her research interests include communication theories, feminist theories, qualitative methods, gender, culture, and identity. She believes that war does strange things.

Dr. Sarah Hochstetler is Assistant Professor of English at Illinois State University. A wide view of her teaching and research makes visible varied interests, ranging from preservice teacher preparation in writing instruction to marked teacher bodies in the secondary classroom. Her current research centers on issues of identity and includes the ways dominant breast cancer rhetorics shape diagnosed women's conceptualization of self, and how breast cancer rhetorics and cultural pressures affect secondary teachers' disclosure of terminal illness. Sarah's scholarship has been published in journals including *The Clearing House, Language Arts Journal of Michigan,* and *Action in Teacher Education.*

Dr. Denise Hooks-Anderson is an Assistant Professor at Saint Louis University School of Medicine in the Department of Community and Family Medicine. As Board Certified Family Physician, she believes that preventative medicine is her primary career focus. Her practice involves helping to improve patients' lives by preventing disease and teaching patients to incorporate healthy lifestyle changes. An advocate for the uninsured, Dr. Hooks-Anderson has worked extensively with her community. Prior to medical school, she received the prestigious National Health Service Corp award, which is given to an individual who desires to work with the uninsured. For six years, she worked at a community health center caring for patients regardless of insurance status. Because of her passion about disease prevention, Dr. Hooks-Anderson has been featured in local and national publications as well as radio and television. She is currently the Medical Accuracy Editor of *The Saint Louis American* newspaper, and she is a past board member of the Missouri Academy of Family Physicians.

Jamie L. Huber, Ph.D. works at Utah State University where she is the program coordinator for the Center for Women and Gender and a Women and Gender Studies lecturer. Jamie works on the development and implementation of gender-focused outreach and co-curricular programs and services. She also teaches core WGS courses at the undergraduate and graduate levels. Her own research focuses on reproductive justice, feminist activism, violence prevention, and the intersections of identities in various women-centered social movements.

Dr. Elise E. Labbé is Professor and Chair of Psychology at the University of South Alabama. She also taught at Virginia Polytechnic Institute and State University and University of Miami. Dr. Labbé received her B.A. in Psychology from Loyola University, New Orleans and M.A. and Ph.D. in Clinical Psychology from Louisiana State University. Dr. Labbé has published over 70 professional, peer-reviewed publications in clinical and health psychology and has presented at over 90, regional, national and international conferences. Dr. Labbé recently published *Psychology Moment by Moment: A Guide to Enhancing Your Clinical Practice with Mindfulness and Meditation*. She teaches undergraduate health psychology and graduates courses in advanced health psychology, and clinical and counseling psychology practicum for the Combined Clinical/Counseling Psychology Doctoral program. She has served as Director of Clinical Training for the Doctoral Program and Director of the Psychological Clinic. She has developed both clinical and research programs on mindfulness and health.

Dr. Pamela J. Lannutti is an Associate Professor and Director of Graduate Programs in Professional and Business Communication in the Department of Communication at La Salle University. She earned her B.A. from LaSalle University (1995) and an M.A. (1997) and Ph.D. (2001) in Communication at the University of Georgia. Dr. Lannutti uses both quantitative and qualitative methods to examine communication in personal relationships. Much of her current research focuses on the legal recognition of same-sex marriage and its impact on same-sex couples, their social networks and communities. She has published over 20 articles in a variety of academic journals, including *Human Communication Research, Communication Studies, Journal of Social and Personal Relationships,* and *Journal of Homosexuality.*

Dr. Edith LeFebvre, PhD, teaches at California State University Sacramento in the Communication Studies Department. She received both her PhD in Rhetoric and Communication and a Master's in Psychology from the University of Oregon. Her areas of specialty are conflict management, persuasion, health communication, political communication, intercultural, interpersonal, public speaking, training and development, and nonverbal communication. She has been active in consulting professional and government organizations throughout her career. She is a certified trainer in mediation and has also served as a community mediator. She has taught at Semester at Sea where she circumnavigated the planet. She has also taught at the International University in Bangkok, Thailand; the University of Oregon; Western Washington University; Lane Community College in Oregon; Consumnes Community College, Sierra Community College, Folsom Lake Community College, and the Center for Continuing Education (the preceding four all located in the Sacramento, California, area).

Dr. Katie Love is an Assistant Professor of Nursing at the University of Saint Joseph and Director of the Multicultural RN-BS program. She has developed the program to focus on understanding oppression, historical discrimination, and disparities. She also mentors these undergraduates in doing community engagement through research, activism, and leadership experiences. Her research focuses on issues of social justice, mutliculturalism, sustainability, holistic health, and community. She is the author of the nursing pedagogy "empowered holistic nursing education," which focuses on creating empowered spaces for healthful learning experiences. Additionally, she volunteers as Director of Sustainability in Health and Wellness at an independent school in Connecticut. This position combines all of her passions, including sustainable and holistic nutrition in a pre-K through 12th-grade setting. She is also a mother to a 2-year-old and twin infant boys.

Dr. Annette Madlock Gatison is an Associate Professor in the Department of Communications at Southern Connecticut State University. She completed her doctoral work in Intercultural Communication and Rhetoric at Howard University in 2007 and is a former Howard University Preparing Future Faculty Fellow. She earned her Master's degree in Communication Studies, a Bachelor's degree in Organizational Studies, and a certificate in Post-Secondary Teaching from Bethel University. Madlock Gatison's current research and writing, The Pink and The Black Project®, focuses on the negotiation of identity and the spiral of silence as it relates to women's health; and on the communicative practices of breast cancer survivors, their family, and their friends.

To ground and inform her research for practical application, Dr. Madlock Gatison is currently serving on the Breast Cancer Consortium Advisory Board; an international partnership committed to the scientific and public discourse about breast cancer; and promotes collaborative initiatives among researchers, advocates, health professionals, educators, and others who focus on the systemic factors that impact breast cancer as an individual experience, a social problem, and a health epidemic. She is also a graduate of the National Breast Cancer Coalitions (NBCC) Project L. E.A. D. (2013), which is an intensive six-day science institute taught by renowned research faculty covering the basics of cancer biology, genetics, epidemiology, research design, and advocacy.

Her book, *Embracing the Pink Identity*, is under contract with Lexington Books and is slated for release. in 2015. Dr. Gatison has presented over 30 papers at various professional conferences. She has also published selections in the SAGE Reference *Encyclopedia of Cancer and Society, 2nd Edition*, edited by Colditz and Golson, 2015 and the SAGE Reference *Multimedia Encyclopedia of Women in Today's World* edited by Strange and Oyster, 2012, among others.

Jennifer Malkowski (M.A., San Diego State University, 2008) is a doctoral candidate in the Department of Communication at the University of Colorado Boulder. Her research focuses on the rhetoric of health and medicine and pays particular attention to how issues of identity, gender, and inequality influence healthcare and policy processes. Most broadly, she examines messages that occur at the political, physician, and patient level to illuminate stages of disease messaging that contribute to public and private understanding of autonomy, risk, and responsibility. Specifically, she employs rhetorical methods of textual analysis to explore tensions between a physician's obligation to safeguard public health and the rights of individuals to make decisions concerning vaccination. In addition to her appointment as an instructor in her home department, Jennifer also serves as a communication coach with the Foundations of Doctoring Program at Anschutz Medical Campus, University of Colorado School of Medicine at Denver.

Dr. Yuping Mao is an Assistant Professor in the Department of Communication Studies at California State University Long Beach. She was recently an Assistant Professor in the Department of Media and Communication at Erasmus University in Rotterdam, the Netherlands. Prior to moving to Europe, Yuping worked as the academic developer in the Graduate Program of Communications and Technology at the University of Alberta in Canada. Her research focuses on intercultural, organizational, and health communication. Yuping teaches undergraduate and graduate courses on research methods, organizational communication, health communication, media campaigns, and culture, new media, and international business. She supervises both undergraduate and graduate theses. Her work has appeared in several peer-reviewed journals and edited books, including *Communication Research, Canadian Journal of Communication, China Media Research, International Journal of Health Planning and Management, Journal of Substance Use,* and *Italian Journal of Pediatrics.*

Dr. Lu Shi is an Assistant Professor in the Department of Public Health Sciences, Clemson University. Previously a research scientist at UCLA School of Public Health, Lu Shi has been developing the microsimulation model to forecast future health trends for the national and state populations. He is also designing the dissemination strategy of research results, using his graduate training and professional experience as a communication expert. Before coming to the United States, he worked for three years as a journalist in China. He has published many peer-reviewed journal articles in disease prevention and early detection, including substance abuse, obesity prevention, health communication, and cancer screening. He is currently running randomized controlled trials of mindfulness-based meditation to explore its cost-effectiveness as a health intervention.

Dr. Carmen Stitt is an Assistant Professor of Communication at California State University, Sacramento. Her expertise centers on health communication, social influence, and mass media, with a particular interest in how people acquire and share health information in mediated environments. She is a Board Member of the UC Davis Cancer Center-Sacramento State Partnership to Reduce Cancer Disparities. She is also a proponent of natural childbirth and midwifery.

Dr. Erika M. Thomas is an Assistant Professor and the Director of Forensics in the Department of Human Communication Studies at California State University, Fullerton. She earned her Ph.D. from the Department of Communication at Wayne State University in December 2011, her Masters of Arts in communication studies from Miami University in Oxford, Ohio in 2008, and her Bachelor of Arts in communication from John Carroll University in 2004. Ms. Thomas's areas of study include rhetorical criticism and theory, and her research interests include the rhetoric of gender, sex, sexuality and the body. Her work has appeared in *Contemporary Argumentation and Debate* and in the collection of essays, edited by Alena Ruggerio, entitled *Media Depictions of Brides, Wives, and Mothers* (2012, Lexington books). This essay is part of her Master's thesis entitled "The Rhetoric of the Modern American Menstrual Taboo," which received the Top Master's Thesis Award from the National Communication Association, Master's Education Division in 2008.

Index